Implementing Clinical Guidelines

a practical guide

EDITED BY

DEBRA HUMPHRIS
AND
PETER LITTLEJOHNS

FOREWORD BY

GENE FEDER

RADCLIFFE MEDICAL PRESS

© 1999 Debra Humphris and Peter Littlejohns

Radcliffe Medical Press Ltd
18 Marcham Road, Abingdon, Oxon OX14 1AA

British Library Cataloguing in Publication Data

A catalogue record for this book is available from the British Library.

ISBN 1 85775 293 7

Typeset by Acorn Bookwork, Salisbury, Wiltshire
Printed and bound by Biddles Ltd, Guildford and King's Lynn

Contents

Foreword

Mrs Nasrudin, the wife of the famous Sufi Mullah, is woken in the dead of night by the sound of someone scrabbling around outside the house. She opens the shutters and sees her husband on his hands and knees in the middle of the road. She asks, 'What are you doing?' 'I dropped the front door keys and am trying to find them', he replies. 'Where did you drop them?' 'Over there', he says pointing to the pavement. 'But then why are you looking in the road?' 'Because the moon is shining here and I can see what I'm doing.'

I was reminded repeatedly of the Mullah's endeavour to find his keys when reading the case studies in this book. First, because keys to effective guidelines implementation are sometimes hard to find and are not always in the most obvious places. Second, because the 'light' of easily collected data may miss or misconstrue the effect of guidelines on clinical practice.

With the advent of clinical governance and the prospect of explicit service standards in primary and secondary care, guidelines are no longer the preserve of the enthusiast. Their effective implementation has become a task for all clinicians and a managerial imperative. But the research industry spawned by clinical guidelines may be less than helpful when trying to implement guidelines on the ground. A guideline programme that works in a randomised controlled trial in East London general practices may be difficult to apply in a medical outpatients department in Northampton.

So this is a timely book, combining a patchwork quilt of guideline implementation case studies, from the Assisting Clinical

Effectiveness (ACE) Programme in South Thames, with an overview and evaluation of the projects. The projects, many of which have found keys to successful implementation – despite controversy about how to define 'success' – are described in sufficient detail to inform other guideline programmes. Even better, explicit lessons from the projects are drawn in the third section of the book which could save time and prevent (some of the) frustration in those embarking on or extending guideline implementation.

The message that emerges again and again is that guidelines do not implement themselves, no matter how well developed or evidence based they are. Moreover, implementation needs to be planned and managed, integrated with the priorities and structure of target organisations, be they general practices, primary care groups, community or acute trusts. Sometimes this is relatively straightforward, often it is not. By telling stories from the ACE programme the contributors cast light on the challenges that we all face and help us find our own keys to improving clinical practice. That is the whole point of guidelines, isn't it?

Gene Feder
Department of General Practice and Primary Care
St Bartholomew's and the Royal London Medical School
Queen Mary and Westfield College
February 1999

Preface

A key priority of the NHS Executive is to ensure that all care provided by the National Health Service is clinically effective. In a succession of White and Green papers, consultation documents and ministerial speeches the NHS Executive has described its policy and the role that organisations and individuals have within it.

A key component is the reliance on evidence-based guidelines to define the expected standard of care against which clinical performance will be assessed. While there is good evidence that guidelines appropriately created, disseminated and implemented can lead to an improvement in patient care, there is also concern that in day-to-day practice this rarely occurs. Considerable efforts have gone into creating a new breed of evidence-based guidelines that combine the best research with professional opinion. There has been less emphasis on ensuring that guidelines are used effectively on a daily basis. This book is based on the Assisting Clinical Effectiveness (ACE) Programme in South Thames. It describes the day-to-day experiences of individuals trying to implement guidelines in a variety of clinical and organisational settings.

This book is not intended to be read from cover to cover but to act as a manual for busy clinicians and managers seeking to improve the care they provide through the application of clinical guidelines. To help in this process it is divided into three sections.

Part 1.
   Provides the background to the approach we have chosen and describes the ACE Programme.

Part 2.
   A series of case studies written by the protagonists themselves.

Part 3.
   Seeks to collate the general lessons learnt and proposes some practical solutions.

We would expect individuals, depending on their background and interest, to skim Part 1, and concentrate on those case studies in Part 2 that relate most closely to their work experience and then to pick up conclusions relevant to them in Part 3.

Implementing guidelines is a multi-disciplinary activity and this guide is therefore aimed at a broad readership including doctors, nurses, professionals allied to medicine and managers in primary and secondary healthcare locations. In order to make it useful on a daily basis the book has been kept deliberately brief. For those who require further information there are references and suggestions for further reading. The ACE Programme is on-going and we would value feedback on any aspect of the guide. Further information is available on the world wide web at *http://www.sghms.ac.uk/phs/hceu/index.htm.*

Debra Humphris
Peter Littlejohns
February 1999

List of contributors

Katy Damaskinidou
Clinical Research Fellow
Pathfinder Mental Health Services NHS Trust

Carol Dumelow
Research Consultant

Nigel Fisher
Consultant Psychiatrist
Pathfinder Mental Health Services NHS Trust

Peggy Freeman
Assistant Director of Nursing and Operational Services
Worthing and Southlands Hospital NHS Trust

Kim Goddard
Audit Co-ordinator
Pathfinder Mental Health Services NHS Trust

Graham Henderson
Consultant in Public Health Medicine
East Surrey Health Authority

Debra Humphris
Director of the ACE Programme
Senior Research Fellow
Health Care Evaluation Unit
St George's Hospital Medical School

Brian James
Clinical Outcomes Co-ordinator
Brighton Health Care NHS Trust IPC Team

Mike Lawes
Chairman
Tunbridge Wells MAAG

Peter Littlejohns
Professor of Public Health and Director
Health Care Evaluation Unit
St George's Hospital Medical School

Carolyn Miller
Head of the Centre for Nursing and Midwifery
University of Brighton

Cerie Nicholas
Leg Ulcer Facilitator
Merton and Sutton Community NHS Trust

Andrew Polmear
Senior Research Fellow
Academic Unit of Primary Care
Trafford Centre for Graduate Medical Education and Research

Annmarie Ruston
Research Fellow in Primary Care
Centre for Health Services Research
University of Kent

Julie Scholes
Senior Lecturer
Centre for Nursing and Midwifery
University of Brighton

Madeleine St Clair
Manager of Clinical Effectiveness
The Princess Royal Hospital
Haywards Heath

Part 1

1

Where do guidelines come from – and why are they so important?

PETER LITTLEJOHNS

Although clinical guidelines are not new, it is only in the last decade that there has been a rapid growth in their production, initially in the USA (Farmer, 1993), but now occurring in the UK (Cluzeau *et al.*, 1997). In the US the surge of interest has been largely prompted by concerns over variations in clinical practice and their resulting impact on the quality, cost and liability of care. As a result, clinical guidelines have been used in various ways

- assisting clinical decision making by patients and practitioners
- educating individuals and groups
- assessing and assuring the quality of care
- guiding allocation of resources for healthcare
- reducing the risk of legal liability for negligent care (Field and Lohr, 1992).

However, the emphasis was on cost containment and guidelines have evolved into integrated care pathways that form the basis of health maintenance organisations' approach to curbing professional variability.

In the UK the emphasis has been different, with the main initiating factors being the expansion of clinical audit in the late 1980s and early 1990s. This approach has led to guidelines being used to define standards, and acting as a quality dimension in the contracting arrangements between commissioners and providers of health. With the recent emphasis on evidence-based medicine and clinical governance (Scally and Donaldson, 1998), clinical guidelines are seen as a potential unifying mechanism. They will bring together the various managerial and professional approaches to improving the quality of care laid out in the government's consultation paper 'A first class service: quality in the new NHS' (*see* Figure 1.1).

The NHS Executive first described its approach to guidelines in 1996 in the document *Clinical Guidelines: using clinical guidelines to improve patient care within the NHS*. Since then the Royal Colleges and other organisations have clarified their position on guidelines. The role of guidelines has been reinforced by becoming the responsibility of the new National Institute for Clinical Excellence described in the White Paper *The New NHS: modern, dependable*. The proposed model is that evidence-based guidelines are to be commissioned from national bodies and Royal Colleges. Before they are recommended to the NHS, their quality will be critically appraised, a process which also assesses whether issues relating to dissemination and implementation have been addressed. The methodology has already been piloted and for the last two years the Health Care Evaluation Unit has undertaken this assessment on behalf of the NHS Executive. So far 24 guidelines have gone through this process (*see* Box 1.1). Further information on guideline appraisal can be found on the Health Care Evaluation Unit website (*http://www.sghms.ac.uk/phs/hceu/index.htm*).

THE NATIONAL INSTITUTE FOR CLINICAL EXCELLENCE (NICE)

A new National Institute for Clinical Excellence will be established to give new coherence and prominence to information about clinical and cost-effectiveness. It will produce and disseminate:

- clinical guidelines based on relevant evidence of clinical and cost-effectiveness
- associated clinical audit methodologies and information on good practice
- in doing so it will bring together work currently undertaken by the many professional organisations in receipt of Department of Health funding for this purpose
- it will work to a programme agreed with and funded from current resources by the Department of Health.

The National Institute's membership will be drawn from the health professions, the NHS, academics, health economists and patient interests. It will need to have access to an appropriate range of skills, including economic and managerial expertise as well as specialist input on specific issues. The Government will consider developing the role and function of the National Institute as it gathers momentum and experience.

Paragraph 7.11–7.12 *The New NHS: modern, dependable*
Cm 3807: December 1997

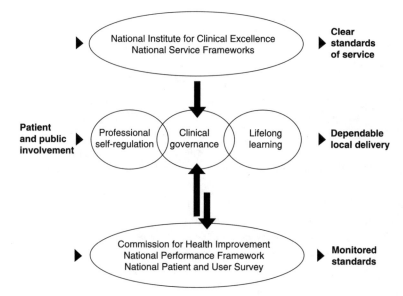

Figure 1.1 The role of clinical guidelines in the government's strategy to improve quality in the NHS. [From: Secretary of State for Health (1998) *A First Class Service: quality in the new NHS.* The Stationery Office, London.]

Box 1.1   Guidelines appraised by the Health Care Evaluation Unit on behalf of the NHS Executive

- Palliative care
- Low back pain
- Chronic critical lower limb ischaemia
- Primary care management of recurrent wheeze in adults
- Primary care management of stable angina
- Upper GI haemorrhage
- Lymphoedema following breast cancer
- Prevention and management of pressure sores
- Care of suicidal patients in A&E
- Speech and language therapy
- Adults with poorly controlled epilepsy
- Primary and out-patient management of groin hernia in adults
- ACE inhibitors in the primary care management of adults with symptomatic heart failure
- The choice of antidepressants for depression in primary care
- Aspirin for the secondary prophylaxis of vascular disease in primary care
- Non-steriodal anti-inflammatory drugs (NSAIDs) versus basic analgesia in the treatment of pain believed to be due to degenerative arthritis
- The primary care management of dementia
- The management of imminent violence in clinical settings
- Initial investigation and management of the infertile couple
- The initial management of menorrhagia
- Strategies to prevent and treat osteoporosis
- Improving the care for patients with malignant cerebral glioma
- The management of menorrhagia in secondary care
- The management of infertility in secondary care

2

How effective are clinical guidelines?

PETER LITTLEJOHNS AND DEBRA HUMPHRIS

With such high expectations, what evidence is there that guidelines can effectively improve patient care. Using Lohr's definition of guidelines as systematically developed statements, which assist in decision making about appropriate healthcare for specific clinical conditions, Grimshaw and Russell undertook a systematic review applying strict methodological criteria (Grimshaw and Russell, 1993). This review has subsequently been updated and has been published as *Effective Health Care Bulletin*, No. 9.

Their conclusion was that specific guidelines do improve clinical practice, when introduced in the context of rigorous evaluations. However, the size of the improvements in performance can vary considerably and significant improvements can only be achieved if guidelines are developed, disseminated and implemented in an appropriate manner. Since then there have been numerous systematic reviews, together with primary quantitative and qualitative research addressing these three areas of activity, although the emphasis has tended to be on the creation of guidelines. Furthermore, much of the research has been centred around randomised controlled trial methodology with specific interventions (e.g. prescribing). This has meant that follow-up assessments have been short term and the generalisability of the results questionable. Very little work has been done to identify the key features of effective guideline dissemination and implementation over a sustained period.

Where do guidelines fit into the other approaches to changing clinical practice?

Encouraging practitioners to incorporate research evidence into daily practice is complex. Identifying the best way has proved so difficult that it has become the subject of research itself. The NHS Research and Development soon realised that if it was to justify spending approximately £1 million a day of NHS funds it would need to demonstrate that the research it supported was being translated into real improvements in patient care. To strengthen the development aspects of the research and development programme a specific research programme was created entitled, 'The evaluation of methods to promote the implementation of research findings'. Under the directorship of Professor Andrew Haines, 20 priority areas were identified. On the first round of bids 32 projects were supported at a cost of £4 million. Guidelines formed a significant part of many of these proposals.

An initial systematic review commissioned by the programme concluded that there were no magic bullets. Since then there have been many attempts to identify effective strategies for bringing about change in professional behaviour. These have ranged from more systematic reviews (now increasing to 20 in the last 7 years), summing the evidence derived only from randomised controlled trials, through to techniques in which practitioners are asked directly what makes them change their practice. These studies have assessed a range of individual techniques as well as various combinations of them:

- continuing medical education

- the role of guidelines

- computerised decision support systems

- one to one transmission of information

- activities of opinion leaders

- the participation of clinicians in trials

- the provision of research-based information to patients

- the role of clinical audit and the feedback of information to practitioners

- whole organisational approaches

- legislation for change.

These approaches can also be classified according to the origins of their theoretical basis (e.g. educational, epidemiological, marketing, behavioural, social interaction, organisational and coercive).

There have been no conclusive results but some general lessons have emerged. As Richard Grol comments, no method is superior (Grol, 1997). Each proposed change in clinical practice needs to be carefully planned; all key protagonists need to be identified as well as the associated barriers. Specifically designed interventions will need to be implemented for each obstacle. The whole process will need to be co-ordinated and progress evaluated.

In general, educational, epidemiological and marketing approaches appear to be particularly effective at the dissemination stage; marketing and social interaction approaches at the adoption phase; behavioural and organisation at the implementation phase; and organisational and coercive approaches to maintain the desired performance. Often a single strategy is not enough; a combination is needed to achieve a lasting effect.

Individuals will perceive differently the implications of these changes. In the literature five characteristics of innovation have been highlighted, each of which may be considered differently by an individual in deciding whether or not to change: relative advantage, compatibility with current beliefs, complexity (although more complex changes may be difficult to initiate they may be longer lasting), observability and trialability (can you see it in action, can you try it out?). This means that selective but integrated strategies will be needed for professionals and the public to address each of these features. Our experience in implementing national and local guidelines supports these findings.

In 1993 the NHS Executive developed a strategic framework for the integration of multi-disciplinary guidelines into the corporate agenda of the local NHS organisations. They had three major strands: the development of individual guidelines based on scientific review and professional consensus; implementation of guidelines in pilot sites and the evaluation of that process; and translation of the national guidelines into local guidelines (or protocols) that were linked to clinical audit and the contracting process. Debra Humphris was responsible for organising the implementation and a number of key features were identified. It was evident that both creating and maintaining the conditions for guideline implementation were active processes that involved the whole organisation.

Preparation is essential

Before any implementation is attempted it is important to show that there is a gap in performance that will motivate clinicians to seek improvements in clinical practice. Clinicians need to think carefully through the process and its implications. The discussion should include patients and commissioners who ultimately have to pick up the costs and consequences of any change. It is only by linking implementation to the corporate plan and priorities of the organisation that changes in practice can be enabled and sustained.

Equally influential are the managerial context and its philosophy; dissonance between these and the implementers' aspirations will lead to considerable tension. Taking time to work through these early on may avoid conflict later. A decision may be made not to implement a guideline at this stage if circumstances do not favour its success.

The general advice now is that local organisations should be seeking to adapt national guidelines rather than starting from scratch. This process should provide an awareness of the broader issues and risks to the organisation at an early stage. If the decision is made to proceed, a plan for implementation should be established that should include clear objectives and a time-scale.

Take time

The emphasis of the implementation on the pilot sites was to take time to develop a reasonable and considered process at a pace that was appropriate locally without allowing it to stall. In one trust an initial force field analysis was carried out to work out the design of the project objectives, criteria for success and time-scale. The abiding lesson is not to underestimate the time required for the whole process: time spent planning will not be wasted.

Clinicians

Clinicians are the real agents of change. Engaging all the appropriate players in the initial process is essential. Increasingly, clinical guidelines have a multi-professional emphasis and impact, and require appropriate inter-professional involvement. The easiest way to promote multi-professional ownership has been by becoming actively involved in existing multi-professional networks. This is important as, like audit, guidelines are likely to reflect the culture of an organisation rather than dictate it.

Education

Implementation provides an opportunity for multi-professional education that is sensitive to local arrangements. This approach ensures ownership and ongoing commitment. Staff will need to be educated about the technical content of the guidelines as well as made aware of the connections with the other quality initiatives within their organisation. Guidelines can form the basis of local continuing professional development that both managers and clinicians consider relevant.

Quality and clinical audit

Linking guideline implementation into an organisation-wide strategic approach to quality and clinical audit assists both processes. Any strategy for implementation of guidelines will reflect professional and managerial cultures; a well-managed implementation process will convey a powerful message of an organisation's commitment to improving quality.

In conclusion, successful guideline implementation requires the understanding that apparently simple and straightforward changes are set within a complex chain of interdependent systems that may block progress. To cause change to occur with the first flush of enthusiasm is not particularly difficult, to make them last is a real challenge.

3

The Assisting Clinical Effectiveness (ACE) Programme

DEBRA HUMPHRIS

The ACE Programme was established by the Health Care Evaluation Unit (HCEU) in 1996 to assist the development of effective clinical practice in South Thames.[1] This was to be achieved through the implementation of clinical guidelines integrated with clinical audit. Invitations to bid for project grants of £30 000 were sent out to all trusts and health authorities in the region. Proposals had to be a joint venture between healthcare providers and purchasers, and all the proposals were to be assessed on the following criteria:

- *improving patient outcomes*

    The area of clinical concern selected should have potential for

---

[1]Initially in South West Thames and then in South Thames, which was the result of South West and South East Thames merging.

improving specific patient outcomes locally and should be agreed by both purchaser and provider before commencement.

- *the quality of clinical guideline*

  The clinical guideline to be implemented must be evidence based and have been endorsed by the appropriate professional organisations.

- *patient involvement*

  Given the area of clinical concern there should be appropriate involvement of users and/or patient organisations in all stages of the process.

- *collaboration*

  Proposals must demonstrate collaborative inter-professional working with active purchaser support and involvement. Consideration must also be given to working across the range of appropriate interfaces.

- *education and support*

  Implementation should take an educational approach providing continuing professional development opportunities.

- *monitoring*

  Criteria derived from the guidelines should form the basis of a related clinical audit programme to monitor changes in practice and improvements in patient outcomes.

There should be a clear management plan and time-scale for the project, including review points and the criteria for success. Support of the chief executives of the organisations involved as well as senior managers and clinicians involved is imperative.

Twenty proposals were submitted and assessed by a panel consisting of managers, public health doctors, clinicians and patient representatives.

Graham Elderfield – Chief Executive, Crawley and Horsham NHS Trust

Dr Brian Fisher – Primary Care Development, LSL Health Commission

Debra Humphris – Senior Research Fellow, HCEU

Dr Marcia Kelson – College of Health

Professor Peter Littlejohns – Director, HCEU

Dr Lois Lodge – Public Health, South Thames NHS Executive

Table 3.1   ACE sites in 1997–98

Site	Guideline topic
Tunbridge Wells MAAG Kent and Sussex Weald NHS Trust Hastings & Rother NHS Trust	The implementation of guidelines for the management of leg ulcers in the community.
Merton & Sutton Community NHS Trust Merton, Sutton & Wandsworth Health Authority	The management of leg ulcers in the community.
Brighton Health Care NHS Trust East Sussex Health Authority	Implementation of the clinical guidelines on the management of menorrhagia.
Eastern Surrey Health Authority East Surrey Healthcare NHS Trust Epsom Healthcare NHS Trust	Implementation of guidelines for referral of patients with breast problems in East Surrey.
Pathfinder Mental Health Services NHS Trust Merton, Sutton & Wandsworth Health Authority	Using clinical guidelines to implement evidence-based practice in the care of people with schizophrenia.
Mid Sussex NHS Trust West Sussex Health Authority	The management of acute, severe asthma.

The project was anticipated to be a collaborative process between the HCEU and each site. Six sites were chosen (Table 3.1) (*see* map, p. ix).

Management of the project

A programme of learning days was provided by the HCEU, with input from appropriate outside speakers, to support the participants with the change process. The programme was based on the principles of implementation and the management of change, rather than the specifics of the guideline's technical content. In addition to this Debra Humphris visited each site and sat in on at least one of each of their steering group meetings. Support was also given to the sites via telephone. Where possible the participants from each of the sites were encouraged to network with and share with each other. The programme leader encouraged sites to connect with other sources of support outside the region.

Learning programme

July 1996 Briefing Day	Welcome and introduction Overview of ACE Programme Consumer involvement in audit and guidelines Critical appraisal of clinical guidelines Managing the change process
October 1996	Review of site progress Research and development: the links with clinical effectiveness Managing change: strategies and methods ACE Programme: evaluation framework
January 1997	Cancelled due to participant's implementation workload
April 1997	Evaluation of progress and lessons learned

Part 2

4

The management of women with menorrhagia

BRIAN JAMES AND ANDREW POLMEAR

Location

This project was undertaken in primary and secondary care in the Brighton area of South Thames. A single trust was involved covering a population of 288 000 patients served by 160 general practitioners.

Background

The Brighton project to improve the management of women with menorrhagia owes its origins to two separate sources. The Department of Gynaecology of Brighton Health Care NHS Trust convened a group to look at the management of dysfunctional uterine bleeding in secondary care. Independently, the Academic Unit of Primary Care at the University of Sussex chose to look at the management of menorrhagia in primary care, as an exercise in the implementation of an evidence-based guideline.

The topic of menorrhagia was chosen for several reasons.

1 It is important.

- 5% of women aged 30–49 consult their GP every year complaining of excessive menstrual loss.
- By the age of 43, 1 in 10 women in the UK has had a hysterectomy, many of them for menorrhagia.

2 Treatment can be effective.

- Five different drugs offer the chance of improvement of between 25% and 95%.
- If drug treatment fails, hysterectomy is 100% successful.
- Endometrial ablation leads to no, or light, bleeding in over three-quarters of women, although with a re-operation rate of up to 23% by 2 years.

3 There is room for improvement in the management of menorrhagia by both GPs and hospital clinicians.

- The drug most commonly prescribed for this condition by GPs, norethisterone, is the least effective, not having been convincingly shown to be better than placebo.
- Dilatation and curretage (D&C) is still performed as part of the work-up for women with menorrhagia, even though the incidence of intrauterine pathology in women under 40 years old is sufficiently uncommon for endometrial sampling to be unnecessary. Women over 40 do need endometrial sampling but less invasive methods are available.
- Past audit projects, both locally and nationally, have indicated that hysterectomy rates vary considerably between clinicians and between hospitals in a way that cannot be explained by differences in the needs of patients.

4 Evidence-based national guidance exists (*Effective Health Care Bulletin: the management of menorrhagia*, August 1995, No. 9).

• This bulletin has strengths and weaknesses as guidance. As a systematic review it is strong; the authors searched for the evidence systematically, appraised it and synthesised it appropriately. The authors went on to propose changes in clinical practice but without the systematic approach necessary for guideline production. The guidance only covered some aspects of the management of menorrhagia. The recommendations were not piloted nor were comments made on its implementation and audit.

From *Effective Health Care Bulletin* the project group chose three criteria for audit. The choice was based on the fact that the criteria focused on the three areas in which the group hoped to change practice; that they were simple; and that their audit was feasible. They were:

1 GPs should offer at least one course of effective drug therapy prior to referral for surgical treatment.

2 D&C should not be performed on women aged under 40, and its use in older women could be replaced by cheaper and safer methods of uterine sampling.

3 Since no management option is superior in all respects, women should be assisted to make informed choices about how to be treated.

The project group was multi-professional, with representation from primary and secondary care, and from several professions within these areas. The group consisted of:

Dr Lisa Argent, GP at Newhaven Medical Centre

Mr Andrew Fish, Consultant in Obstetrics and Gynaecology (project leader)

Mr Brian James, Clinical Outcomes Co-ordinator (project facilitator)

Dr Andrew Polmear, Senior Research Fellow, The Trafford Centre, University of Sussex

Ms Vi Simpson, Gynaecology Outpatients Clerk

Ms Jackie Stevenson, GP Practice Nurse

We also had direct input from the following clinicians:

Dr Saikat Bannerjee, Gynaecology SHO

Dr John Bidmead, Gynaecology Registrar

Ms Annette Keen, Head of Nursing (Gynaecology)

Methods

The methods used for the implementation and audit of the guideline varied according to the criterion under study.

Criterion 1   GPs should offer at least one course of effective drug therapy prior to referral for surgical treatment

This was an unashamedly top-down implementation. Enquiry of individual GPs revealed no memory of the *Effective Health Care Bulletin* even though it had been sent to GPs the year before. GPs did not sense that norethisterone was ineffective, nor did they know that its use was unsupported by the evidence.

Baseline data were obtained by analysing GPs referral letters for menorrhagia to the gynaecology clinic from 1 February 1996 to 30 June 1996. The intervention was then begun with an education session at the local postgraduate medical centre, to which all GPs in the Brighton, Hove and Lewes area were invited, as well as all medical staff in gynaecology.

The education session took place on 11 July 1996 and involved presentations of the evidence from the bulletin to participants. The evidence was presented from the viewpoint of a GP (by Andrew Polmear) and current practice from the viewpoint of the specialist (by Andrew Fish). The method chosen was to take the audience through a series of stages, from initial satisfaction with current management, to scepticism about the guideline, to reluctant agreement with the guideline, to enthusiasm at the prospect of more effective treatment. Most of the GPs were known personally to Andrew Polmear and Andrew Fish, and the session scored high marks for relevance, content and presentation. The audience were given the opportunity to comment on the evidence, and to alter the guideline if they wished; none did. The GPs in the audience were asked if they agreed that their referral letters should be monitored for adherence to the guideline and that they should receive feedback on the results of the analysis. There were no dissenters.

All 160 GPs in the area, whether they had attended the session or not, received a letter summarising the session. Again, permission was asked from those who had not attended the session, to audit their referral letters and to give them feedback on the extent to which their referrals met the criterion. Those GPs who agreed to receive feedback on the overall compliance of referrals with the guideline received further letters at 3 and at 6 months, reminding them of the guideline and giving information on the number of referrals conforming to it.

Criterion 2   D&C should not be performed on women aged under 40, and its use in older women could be replaced by cheaper and safer methods of uterine sampling

This part of the study also used a before and after approach, with data on the number of D&Cs performed being collected before and after the introduction of the guideline. For the baseline sample, data were already available on all women who had been referred to Brighton Health Care in the financial year 1994–95. The project group decided to use these data, comparing them with data on women referred to Brighton Health Care immediately after the guideline had been introduced. For the first set of women, data were taken from the patients' records and recorded on a data collection sheet. For the second set, data were recorded at the time of the first consultation by the consultant gynaecologist. The data collection sheet included details of the treatment given in primary care and the investigations and treatment planned in secondary care. Once the patients' treatment was completed, the case notes were examined to extract information on what management the patient had received. The data collection forms were scanned using Teleform character recognition software, and the results analysed using SPSS statistical analysis package.

Criterion 3   Since no management option is superior in all respects, women should be assisted to make informed choices about how to be treated

Interviews were performed on a sample of women who had undergone a hysterectomy, to discover whether, in their perception, they were assisted to make an informed choice. The practice nurse was selected to conduct these interviews because she had previous experience of interviewing patients, was clinically trained (and therefore able to answer any questions women may ask) and also because it was felt that patients might feel more comfortable discussing this subject with another woman, especially one who was not part of the hospital team about which the patient was being asked to comment.

Patients undergoing hysterectomy for menorrhagia were sent a letter asking them if they would consent to being interviewed, and they were given the choice of being interviewed at home or at the hospital. Each interview lasted for about 1 hour. The interview schedule was based around the experiences women had during their treatment, whether they felt they had been involved in making decisions and how they felt about the way those decisions had been made.

Results

Criterion 1

The intervention began with the meeting on 11 July 1996. The subsequent mailing was on 12 July. Twenty-two GPs attended the education session out of a possible 160. All agreed to receive details of the audit. A further 37 responded to the subsequent letter inviting them to receive feedback, making a total of 59.

Two methods for assessing the effect of the intervention were used.

1 *Prescribing data for the Brighton area*

The guideline suggested that norethisterone is not an effective treatment for menorrhagia. Of drugs that have been shown to be effective, tranexamic acid is one of the more effective with few side-effects. Unlike norethisterone, it has almost no role other than the treatment of menorrhagia. A fall in norethisterone prescribing might or might not be due to more appropriate prescribing in menorrhagia. A rise in the use of tranexamic acid would be a strong indication of more effective prescribing.

(a) *Norethisterone.* Norethisterone prescribing rose over the 6 months before the intervention (from 248 items in January 1996 to 359 items in July 1996 – the month of the intervention.) Norethisterone prescribing then fell over the 6 months after the intervention (from 359 to 219) (*see* Figure 4.1).

It is tempting to postulate that the intervention caused the change seen from July onwards. However, prescribing data from Eastbourne (*see* Figure 4.2) show a similar rise to a peak in July followed by a fall, although the rise and fall are less marked. This suggests that some other factor was responsible for some of the prescribing changes seen in Brighton, although not necessarily all of them. This factor may be the use of norethisterone to postpone a period during the holiday months of May to August. Prescribing data for 1995 show a similar seasonal change.

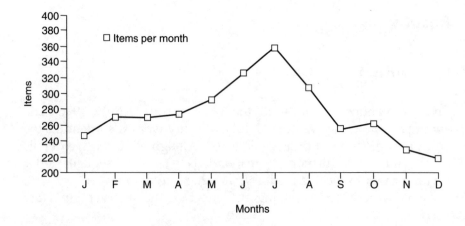

Figure 4.1 Norethisterone prescribing in Brighton in 1996.

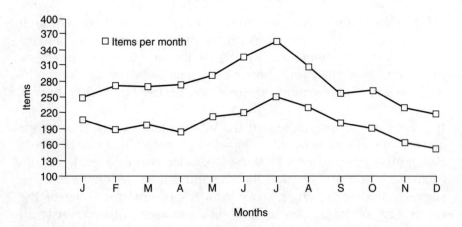

Figure 4.2 Norethisterone prescribing in Brighton (upper line) and Eastbourne (lower line) in 1996.

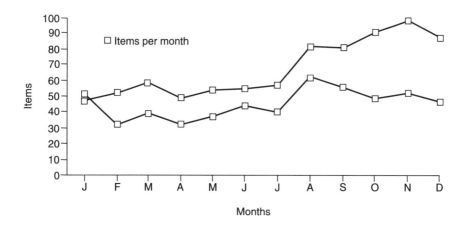

Figure 4.3 Tranexamic acid prescribing in Brighton (upper line) and Eastbourne (lower line) in 1996.

(b) *Tranexamic acid.* Prescribing data for Brighton and Eastbourne for tranexamic acid showed that the prescription of tranexamic acid increased from 47 for a month to a high of 99 in Brighton. In Eastbourne there was no overall rise in tranexamic prescriptions (*see* Figure 4.3). Statistical analysis was performed by taking the change in the number of items prescribed in Brighton for each month of 1996 compared with the same month in 1995, and comparing the mean of these changes to the mean of the changes in Eastbourne calculated in the same way. The difference between the two areas is significant ($p = 0.016$). The intervention is a possible explanation for this difference.

2 *Analysis of GP referrals*

GP referral letters from February 1996 to March 1997 were marked by members of the project group against the criterion. Forty of the 103 GP referral letters analysed failed to mention whether any drugs had been given before referral. On the

Table 4.1   Number of referral letters meeting the criterion

Period	All GPs	GPs requesting feedback	GPs not requesting feedback
1996			
Feb–June	11 out of 33	1 out of 8	10 out of 25
Intervention:			
11 July 1996			
July–Sept	11 out of 29	3 out of 5	8 out of 24
Oct–Dec	4 out of 15	3 out of 7	1 out of 8
1997			
Jan–Mar	5 out of 26	3 out of 9	2 out of 17

assumption that these patients had not received an effective drug (the worst-case scenario) there was no overall improvement in GPs' compliance with the guideline. GPs who agreed to receive feedback did improve their performance dramatically, followed by gradual decline, although the numbers are too small for statistical significance. The performance of GPs who did not attend the meeting nor agree to receive feedback appears to have worsened during the same period (*see* Table 4.1.)

This table raises the possibility that the decision to receive feedback and receiving that feedback improved GPs' prescribing, even if the effect seems to decline with time. However, the apparent deterioration in the performance of the group who did not receive feedback is unexpected. If the intervention affected the performance of those GPs adversely, for instance by making them resistant to the message of the project, then the overall benefit to patients is reduced or nullified.

Criterion 2

Although in England in 1993–94, 106 146 D&Cs were performed, the Gynaecology Department of Brighton Health Care does not

Table 4.2   Rate of D&Cs

	Pre-guidelines	Post-guidelines
Number of D&Cs for menorrhagia in 1 year	1	0
Total women referred with menorrhagia	33	48

appear to have been contributing to this number, even in women aged over 40. There was therefore no room for improvement.

Table 4.2 shows the D&C rate before and after the introduction of the guidelines.

Criterion 3

1 *Hysterectomy rate*

The percentage of women referred for menorrhagia who underwent or who were put on the waiting list for hysterectomy fell from 39% before the guideline was introduced to 12% after its introduction. There was so much discussion nationally about the overuse of hysterectomy that this change cannot be attributed to the guideline. Indeed, a reduction in the hysterectomy rate was not included in the guideline.

Table 4.3 shows the number of hysterectomies performed for menorrhagia before and after the introduction of the guidelines.

Table 4.3   Number of hysterectomies

	Pre-guidelines	Post-guidelines
Number	11	3
Total women referred	33	48

Table 4.4   Number on waiting list for hysterectomy

	Pre-guidelines	Post-guidelines
Number	2	3
Total women referred	33	48

As the waiting list for non-urgent hysterectomy was over one year, the number of women on the waiting list for hysterectomy was also recorded in Table 4.4, which shows the number of women on the waiting list for hysterectomy for menorrhagia before and after the introduction of the guidelines.

2 *Interview of patients after hysterectomy*
Five women referred for hysterectomy in 1994–95 were interviewed using a semi-structured approach. The relevant results were as follows.

• All women were expecting a hysterectomy before they came to hospital.

• All women were advised they might have a hysterectomy by their GP.

• All those interviewed were unable to recall the exact details of their past treatment for menorrhagia.

• In two cases, the patient felt that the hospital consultant had made the decision that she should have a hysterectomy. In the remaining cases, the patient felt she had been involved in the decision.

• In all cases, the women were happy with who made the decision.

• All women interviewed would have liked to have talked to someone post-operatively to discuss issues raised by having had a hysterectomy, especially to discuss sexual issues.

These findings raise three issues:

1 Women's expectations of whether they will have a hysterectomy for menorrhagia are formed before their first contact with the

hospital service. The GP is important in the formation of those expectations. Any attempt to change the treatment in secondary care must involve GPs so that they can prepare patients appropriately for what they might expect when they reach hospital.

2 Women were satisfied with the way the decision about hyster-ectomy was made, regardless of who made it. This seems to conflict with the recommendation of *Effective Health Care* that women should be assisted to make their own decisions. Re-examination of the bulletin reveals that the recommendation was not evidence based, but rather an opinion of the authors. Because of this the project team agreed that further interviews of women against this criterion were not justified.

3 Women need more counselling about the effects of hysterectomy on their personal life, and they want this, not in order to assist their decision making, but to help them to know what to expect post-operatively. This has implications for the delivery of a service to women undergoing hysterectomy.

Discussion and further inquiry

The project group felt that there was evidence that the intervention had made a difference to GP prescribing; and that, even if it had not influenced management in secondary care, useful lessons about what patients really want had been learned.

In order to explore what aspects of the primary care element of the intervention had made it effective, we sent a questionnaire to the 59 GPs who had agreed to receive feedback. They were asked to give a score, anonymously, for whether the project had had an effect on their prescribing and, if it had, to score seven aspects of the intervention from 1 to 5 where:

- 1 is 'no effect at all',
- 2 is 'a slight effect'
- 3 is 'a moderate effect'
- 4 is 'a substantial effect'
- 5 is 'a great effect'.

They were asked: do you think that this project has had an effect on your prescribing for menorrhagia?

If there was some effect, to what extent do you think the following factors played a part? (Figure 4.4, Q1)

- The source of the message – the *Effective Health Care Bulletin?* (Q2)

- The people who passed on the message – Andrew Fish and Andrew Polmear? (Q3)

- The meeting, if you went to it? (Q4)

- The written material you received initially giving the message above? (Q5)

- The fact that you were part of an audit? (Q6)

- The repetition of the message via the reminders? (Q7)

- The results contained in those reminders? (Q8)

Fifty-five replies were received from 59 GPs, of whom four were unable to comment because of leave or retirement. Only one respondent replied that the project had had no effect on his or her prescribing. The others scored the effect from 2 to 5, with a mean of 3.6. Scores for the aspects of the intervention are shown in Figure 4.4.

Several points of interest emerge.

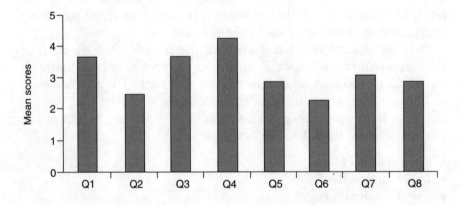

Figure 4.4 Responses to the 'effectiveness' questionnaire.

1 All aspects of the intervention were thought to have had some effect, supporting the idea that a 'scatter gun' approach is likely to produce the largest effect.

2 The aspects thought to have been most beneficial are those of a local and personal nature; namely, the meeting, the identity of the people fronting the project and the personal reminder letters. The factors that had the least effect were that the guideline was national and evidence based, that they were part of an audit and the results of that audit. This is in keeping with other work on the effectiveness of interventions, with the one exception that the lectures were considered useful (see below).

3 The aspect of the intervention that scored highest was the meeting, which took the form of two lectures, albeit with questions at the end. Other work has shown little or no effect from lectures on clinical practice. The project group felt that certain aspects of the meeting, the fact that the speakers were local 'opinion leaders', and that the material was presented in a humorous and personal way, accounted for this.

Other factors that may have facilitated the project were as follows.

• The simplicity of the criteria. They were easy for clinicians to understand and easy for the project group to monitor.

• The project group was supported throughout the project by the Health Care Evaluation Unit of St George's Hospital Medical School. The two members of the group (Brian James and Andrew Polmear) who attended meetings at St George's felt motivated by them and felt that that motivation cascaded down to other members of the group.

Several lessons were learned in the course of the work.

• There is no possibility of benefit from a project aimed at a problem that has already been solved (D&Cs for menorrhagia in Brighton).

• Data collection is time consuming. The project team would now double the time they allow for data collection for future projects.

- Enrolling patients to participate in interviews is difficult and should begin as soon as possible. The response rate in this project was low and could be due to one or more of the following factors:
  - the transient population in the study area
  - the emotional associations with hysterectomy
  - the time that had elapsed since the treatment.

When the methods of qualitative research, in this case interviewing women about their feelings about hysterectomy, are used, the results may be quite different from those expected; indeed, as in this case, they may lead to a questioning of the original assumptions behind the audit. The project group sees this as the strength of this approach.

5

Care of people with schizophrenia

KIM GODDARD, NIGEL FISHER AND KATY DAMASKINIDOU

Location

This project was based in Pathfinder Mental Health Services NHS Trust. The trust provides a comprehensive range of mental health services to the adult population of the outer London Borough of Merton and most of the inner London Borough of Wandsworth. Services are provided predominantly by Community Mental Health Teams (CMHTs). The trust also provides local tertiary services, such as rehabilitation and continuing care services, and national specialist services, such as those for the deaf. The consultant led CMHTs are catchment area based and fully aligned with GP practices. They are organised into well-established multi-disciplinary teams and committed to prioritising the long-term mentally ill. This patient group makes up 70% of community psychiatric nurse (CPN) caseloads. The local service has been judged to work to a high standard by the London Mental Health Taskforce.

Background

Management of people with long-term, severe mental illness continues to cause professional, public and political concern. This reflects the high individual and social morbidity and mortality of these disorders. Although the term 'long-term severe mental illness' covers a wide range of problems, schizophrenia is the most common disorder, with between 3 and 4 per thousand of the general population experiencing problems associated with schizophrenia at any one time.

Whilst there is considerable disagreement on how services should be organised and delivered, there is less dissent about the value of specific interventions. Effective interventions for people with schizophrenia have been detailed by Conway *et al.* (1994). These include behavioural–cognitive therapy for psychotic symptoms, family problem solving therapy, medication (especially the use of atypical antipsychotics such as clozapine) and educational programmes.

The report of the Clinical Standards Advisory Group (CSAG) (1995) on schizophrenia found that the availability of these services was limited in all districts studied. In two of the districts no such services existed at all. One reason for this was a lack of trained staff, although another was a failure to target the severely mentally ill. In the case of atypical antipsychotic medication, where guidelines do commonly exist, these aim to limit the prescribing of the drug on cost grounds alone rather than promoting cost-effective use. The CSAG report confirmed that explicit budgetary limits existed in most districts.

The impetus for this project came from a recent local clinical audit (Plumb and Jeffries, 1996). A senior registrar and a mental health nurse looked at the extent to which two Pathfinder CMHTs met CSAG guidelines in delivering a range of evidence-based interventions for people with schizophrenia. The audit found that in only 4 out of 105 cases audited was there case note evidence to indicate that family work had been considered. Discussion of long-term side-effects of medication was recorded in 7 cases. Only 4 people were receiving the atypical antipsychotic, clozapine, a smaller number than could be expected to benefit from the drug. Interestingly, in the area where there was a clear trust policy and associated guidance, namely the use of the Care Programme Approach (CPA), the audit standards were met in almost 100% of cases. Unlike the clinical interventions, the evidence to support the value of the CPA is controversial.

A simple case note audit is not able to detect what was considered or discussed by clinicians but not entered in the notes. It was evident from discussions with clinicians that there was considerable consensus on what good practice should be. There was less clarity on how to ensure the routine consideration of this practice as applied to individual patients and on identifying clinicians with the skills to implement it.

The project

This project aimed to attempt to make nationally agreed guidelines and standards available and accessible to services in their day-to-day clinical practice. Having received funding from the ACE initiative a project team consisting of a psychiatrist, clinical audit co-ordinator and a research nurse (later succeeded by a research psychiatrist) was established. This group was supported by a service user, pharmacist and a clinical psychologist.

As the starting point, the standards set by the CSAG report were reviewed. These included:

- regular assessment and care for physical ill health

- regular review and monitoring of medication by skilled practitioners

- access to medication shown to be beneficial for people who are otherwise treatment-resistant (e.g. clozapine)

- regular multi-disciplinary review

- a full range of cognitive and behavioural therapies is offered for the relief and self-management of distressing symptoms, impaired functioning and adverse self-attitude

- specific family interventions aimed at relapse prevention

- information and education is provided aimed at recognising and preventing the risk of relapse in those living alone.

Some of these interventions overlap and some, to be implemented in full, would have been beyond the scope of this project. Consequently, we focused on three areas:

- use of the new antipsychotics

- family interventions

- the place of regular physical health checks and screening programmes.

While the CSAG report set standards, these were not supported by specific guidance on how these standards might be achieved. Furthermore, it became apparent that there were neither national nor local guidelines on these areas. Our first task, then, was to develop guidelines that would be acceptable and accessible to the local services.

Method

In attempting to develop the guideline we followed an evidence-based medicine (EBM) approach. The key elements of EBM have been documented elsewhere (Sackett *et al.*, 1997) and include:

(i)   forming answerable clinical questions

(ii)   searching the best external evidence

(iii)   critically appraising the evidence for its validity

(iv)   applying the results locally

(v)   developing an evaluation system for clinical practice.

Critically appraising the evidence

The patient group targeted were those people with a primary diagnosis of schizophrenia, who had persistent symptoms or functional impairment and who had an illness history of at least two years. The applicability of the EBM process to each of the previously audited areas is described below, starting with the relevant clinical question.

Drug intervention

Would the use of an atypical antipsychotic reduce symptoms or side-effects? If so which atypical should be used?
Electronic searches of Medline, PsychLit and the Cochrane Library were completed. Only double-blind randomised controlled trials, published in peer review journals were considered. This yielded a surprisingly small number of references: 13 for clozapine, 6 for risperidone, 3 for olanzapine and none for sertindole. Similar outcome measures were used in most papers (e.g. the Brief Psychiatric Rating Scale) which allowed comparisons to be made in the form of numbers needed to treat (NNTs).[1] Unfortunately, a range of measures were used to evaluate side-effects making comparisons in terms of NNTs beyond the scope of this project. The relevance of these studies to our patients was harder to judge. All the studies had recruited patients with a wide range of illness severity and duration. Disappointingly, no studies compared one atypical antipsychotic against another. Despite this, it was possible to draw some conclusions. There was good evidence that clozapine was superior to conventional antipsychotics (NNTs 3–4). The evidence for the superiority of olanzapine and resperidone was similar but less clear-cut with NNTs ranging from 3 to 15. By our criteria there was no published evidence to support the use of sertindole.

---

[1] The NNT represents the number needed to treat with the new therapy to cause one additional good outcome (e.g. reduction of psychotic symptoms) or prevent one from developing a bad outcome (e.g. extrapyramidal side-effects).

Psychosocial interventions

Would family therapy reduce symptoms or improve function. If so which form of family therapy should be used?
The size and complexity of the literature meant that a systematic review of this field would have been beyond the resources of this locally based project. However, there was a recent systematic review published in the Cochrane Library (Mari and Streiner, 1996). This review confirmed the efficacy of family therapy in terms of reducing relapse rate (NNTs 2–7). The studies involved multiple interventions and the nature of the family therapy varied from study to study. All required practitioners to have some specialist training. Within our services such training is scarce, with the result that it was hard to know how best to advise CMHTs on what the most effective and locally feasible interventions might be. However, advice on future training priorities could be given.

Physical healthcare

Does regular primary healthcare screening reduce physical morbidity in this patient group?
The high physical morbidity and mortality of people with schizophrenia has led some to recommend screening for respiratory and cardiovascular problems in this population at the primary healthcare level (Kendrick, 1996). A small separate survey (Henning, 1997) of patient take-up of health checks locally suggested that this was minimal. Strategies to encourage patient attendance and to liaise on this matter with GPs were rarely reflected in care plans. Discrepancies existed between mental health professionals and patients in the perceived help required for physical health problems. Sadly, despite the indications of this survey, we could identify no randomised controlled trials to support a strategy to improve take-up of healthcare screening in our patient group. As a result, any guidance on this area could not be informed by outcome studies.

As can be seen, the usefulness of EBM varied with the clinical question. The evidence is summarised in Table 5.1.

Table 5.1   Usefulness of EBM

Steps in evidence-based medicine process	Intervention		
	Use of atypical antipsychotics	Family therapy	Primary healthcare screening
Able to set answerable clinical question	✓	✓	✓
Searching for the evidence			
Peer-reviewed, RCTs	✓	✓	✓
Systematic reviews	× *	✓	×
Appraisal of papers for validity and importance			
Relevant patient group	Qualified ✓	Qualified ✓	n/a
Outcome measures	✓	Varied	n/a
Side-effects	×	×	n/a
Cost effectiveness	×	×	n/a
Able to calculate NNTs	✓	✓	n/a
Intervention locally applicable	✓	Qualified	n/a
Able to inform local guideline?	Yes	Only in a limited way	No
Development of evaluation system	Possible	Possible	Possible

*Not available at the time of searching the evidence (January 1997).

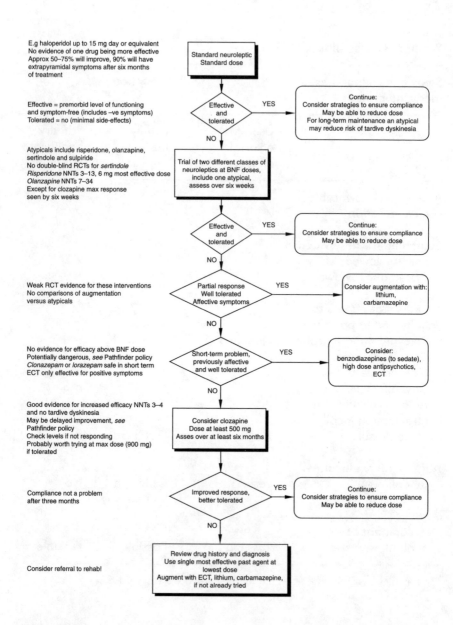

E.g haloperidol up to 15 mg day or equivalent
No evidence of one drug being more effective
Approx 50–75% will improve, 90% will have
extrapyramidal symptoms after six months
of treatment

**Standard neuroleptic
Standard dose**

Effective = premorbid level of functioning
and symptom-free (includes –ve symptoms)
Tolerated = no (minimal side-effects)

**Effective
and
tolerated** — YES → Continue:
Consider strategies to ensure compliance
May be able to reduce dose
For long-term maintenance an atypical
may reduce risk of tardive dyskinesia

NO

Atypicals include risperidone, olanzapine,
sertindole and sulpiride
No double-blind RCTs for *sertindole*
Risperidone NNTs 3–13, 6 mg most effective dose
Olanzapine NNTs 7–34
Except for clozapine max response
seen by six weeks

**Trial of two different classes of
neuroleptics at BNF doses,
include one atypical,
assess over six weeks**

**Effective
and
tolerated** — YES → Continue:
Consider strategies to ensure compliance
May be able to reduce dose

NO

Weak RCT evidence for these interventions
No comparisons of augmentation
versus atypicals

**Partial response
Well tolerated
Affective symptoms** — YES → Consider augmentation with:
lithium,
carbamazepine

NO

No evidence for efficacy above BNF dose
Potentially dangerous, *see* Pathfinder policy
Clonazepam or *lorazepam* safe in short term
ECT only effective for positive symptoms

**Short-term problem,
previously affective
and well tolerated** — YES → Consider:
benzodiazepines (to sedate),
high dose antipsychotics,
ECT

NO

Good evidence for increased efficacy NNTs 3–4
and no tardive dyskinesia
May be delayed improvement, *see*
Pathfinder policy
Check levels if not responding
Probably worth trying at max dose (900 mg)
if tolerated

**Consider clozapine
Dose at least 500 mg
Asses over at least six months**

Compliance not a problem
after three months

**Improved response,
better tolerated** — YES → Continue:
Consider strategies to ensure compliance
May be able to reduce dose

NO

Consider referral to rehab!

**Review drug history and diagnosis
Use single most effective past agent at
lowest dose
Augment with ECT, lithium, carbamazepine,
if not already tried**

Figure 5.1 Draft algorithm for use of neuroleptics in people with schizophrenia. [Much of this algorithm has been derived from *Bethlem and Maudsley Prescribing Guidelines* (3e).]

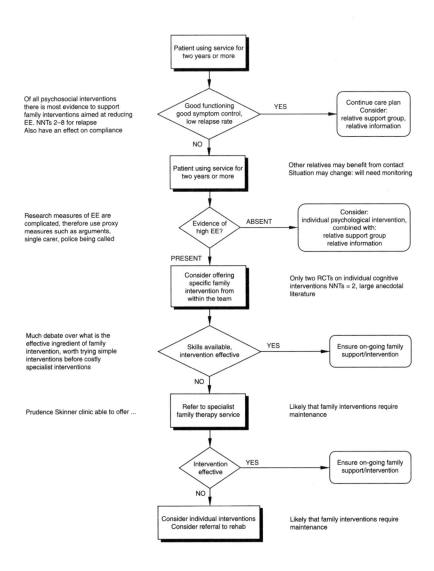

Figure 5.2 Draft algorithm for psychosocial interventions for people with schizophrenia.

Applying the guidelines locally

Our evidence was now more easily scanned, but the problem was how to present it as a locally applicable guideline in an easily digestible form to hard-bitten clinicians? We settled on an algorithm (*see* Figures 5.1 and 5.2) because of its visual impact and intuitive qualities. Local adaptation to the working practices of individual teams could be accommodated by altering the sequence, but not content, of the 'source' algorithm. The accessibility of a guideline is important in its success (Grimshaw and Russell, 1994). Our aim was to produce something that could be reproduced on one sheet of paper and included the strength of evidence for each stage of the guideline. This could then be adapted by each team to produce a checklist to sign-off when an intervention was used. This checklist in effect became the guideline and would double as a monitoring tool. The initial algorithms, as reproduced in Figures 5.1 and 5.2, were annotated by information from the literature reviews.

Education support

Our original project proposal included some ambitious plans for an educational programme. At the same time we knew that high profile attempts to change clinical practice could engender irritation rather than enthusiasm. We settled on an approach that we hoped balanced teaching and involvement. Initial contact with each team was made via one of their regular business meetings. The project team asked for 30 minutes to give some background to the project and to introduce the algorithms. The rest of the time was given up to discussion. Copies of the algorithm were distributed and (perhaps anticipating that for some of the more cynical clinicians only primary sources would satisfy) an evidence pack containing all of the key papers used was produced for each team.

At the end of the session it was suggested that a member of the project team meet two of the team to look in more detail at how the algorithms might be applicable to their patients and how their use could be incorporated into their routine practice. Ideally, we tried to ensure that one of the pair be a senior clinician so that some collaboration and leadership could be established quickly. We were also

Table 5.2 Wimbledon CMHT schizophrenia treatment guideline

This checklist provides prompts for pharmacological and psychosocial interventions for people with schizophrenia. It should be completed by the key worker in conjunction with other relevant disciplines every 6 months or at each care plan review (whichever comes first). A copy should be kept with the care plan in the multi-disciplinary notes. This checklist should be used when reviewing the care of all patients with schizophrenia who have been ill for 2 years or more.

Patient's name: DOB: Date:

Over the past 6 *months*:
1   Has the patient had positive symptoms?   YES/NO
2   Has the patient had negative symptoms?   YES/NO
3   Has the patient had symptoms of depression?   YES/NO

If the answer is YES to any of the above:
4   Do the symptoms impair social functioning
    in any way?   YES/NO
5   If pt has positive symptoms is he/she
    compliant to medication?   YES/NO

If pt has positive and/or negative symptoms:
6   Has a psychosocial intervention been tried?   YES/NO
    Specify (what it was and what was the outcome):

7   Is there evidence of High EE?   YES/NO
8   Has an intervention been considered?   YES/NO
    If YES specify: _____
9   Has an atypical antipsychotic been tried?   YES/NO
    Specify (what it was and what was the outcome):

10 Has a living skills intervention been tried?   YES/NO
    Specify (what it was and what was the outcome):

11 If pt has symptoms of depression has an
    antidepressant been tried?   YES/NO

12 If an atypical antipsychotic was prescribed has the dose been
    increased after 6 weeks?   YES/NO

13 Has there been a trial of 6 further weeks
    on the increased dose of atypical antipsychotic?   YES/NO
14 Has a living skills intervention been tried again?   YES/NO
    Specify (what it was and what was the outcome):

**If the above interventions have been applied and the pt still
has positive and/or negative symptoms:**
15 Has clozapine been considered?   YES/NO
    Has clozapine been tried?   YES/NO
16 Has clozapine been excluded?   YES/NO
    If YES why? Specify: _____

17 If pt had been on depot injection before starting
    on the new antipsychotic has pt been compliant
    with medication?   YES/NO

18 Has a scale been used to measure symptoms
    and/or side-effects?   YES/NO
    Specify: **BPRS   AIMS   HoNOS**   Other: _____

19 Was a physical health check carried out in the
    last year?   YES/NO

Any other comments or suggestions for further interventions?

This checklist was completed by _____

This checklist has been designed by the Wimbledon CMHT and the Assisting
Clinical Effectiveness (ACE) Schizophrenia Guidelines group. Any comments or
queries should be directed to Dr Rozewicz (Consultant Psychiatrist, Wimbledon
CMHT 0181 544 9799) or/and Dr Damaskinidou (Rehab team, SPH ext: 42336)

aware that to continue to be used the guideline had to be workable,
so the input of more than one discipline and grade was important
in sorting out what was practically, and again routinely, possible.
   The second, more intimate, meeting took an individual patient's

case as its starting point. The pair of team members were asked, for example, how they would normally decide on a particular drug treatment, at what point would its use be reviewed and by what criteria? When would they consider family therapy? By following a similar line of discussion it became clear where practice diverged in substance from the guideline and where it diverged only in administrative detail. Where there was a practice difference, the team was reminded of the evidence. This discussion formed the basis of the monitoring checklist (*see* Table 5.2) which, after the meeting, we typed for the team and returned it to them for final comments. In each case we asked that teams include a copy of the checklist in each set of case notes and complete it at their normal patient review meetings. We explained that the checklist would be used by us to audit the extent to which the guidelines were being used at the end of the project and could then be used subsequently by teams to continue the monitoring process.

Results

The success or otherwise of the project could be judged in two ways. First, the extent to which services accepted and adopted the guidelines, and secondly the extent to which the guidelines affected clinical practice in relation to individual patients.

At the time of writing, the process for developing the guidelines had been enthusiastically adopted by two CMHTs, a large general practice and two specialist services. The process of developing the guidelines in the context of each team's own view of good practice and dummy running the checklists with specific patients clearly facilitated this process. The guidelines were truly locally owned. In the longer term and of greater impact is a guideline for the use of new antipsychotics (*see* Figure 5.3) that came out of the above process. This has been adopted by the trust's Drug and Therapeutics Committee and by the host health authority. In contrast to the previous policy, the guideline aims to facilitate the use of the most effective drug rather than imposing financial restrictions.

At present it is not possible to report on the extent to which practice with individual patients has been affected. We are

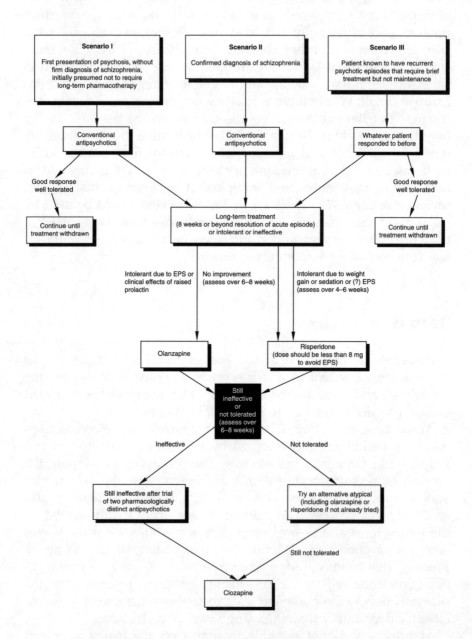

Figure 5.3 Draft algorithm for use of antipsychotic drugs.

currently in the process of re-examining the notes of the patients included in the original audit.

Discussion

The seeming simplicity of the method described above hides problems both foreseen and unimagined. In retrospect, our project was too large, as first proposed, for the time and resources at hand. Mental health services for the severely mentally ill work to a long time-frame – a year is not long for changes to circulate around the system for each patient. Moreover, some interventions themselves, notably family interventions, may take 18 months to 2 years for a measurable improvement in relapse rates to occur (Mari and Streiner, 1996). A survey of staff training and skills (Hayes, 1997) confirmed our expectation that staff having specialist training in family therapy of any form were scarce; although during the life-time of the project a diploma course incorporating basic family work was introduced for CPNs, it will take time for these skills to become widespread. We have no reason to suspect that Pathfinder is unique in these skills being in short supply, rather this reflects a national situation where mental health staff training is changing in response to changing modes of service delivery.

Two key administrative problems occurred that we were unable to foresee. The two CMHTs that we originally planned to work with metamorphosed into one team with a new consultant psychiatrist and several new staff after the project was initiated. This again reflects rapid changes that are occurring in mental health services and was a situation we were unable to predict at the time of planning the project. The result was that some ground had to be re-covered and collaboration re-sought. In addition, a shortage of clinical staff in London meant that it was difficult to recruit a replacement of sufficient knowledge and seniority when our original principal project worker left to seek promotion. Progress was delayed for some months until we were able to recruit a part-time research registrar (KD).

Our key difficulty, however, was that the original standards chosen were not related to any operationalised clinical guideline.

Much of the project resource was thus spent in developing the guidelines themselves. This had its advantages as, whilst the guidelines were not as comprehensive as some that have been produced (American Psychiatric Association, 1997), they were locally owned and, by being brief, could be used in practice. The EBM framework was invaluable to the project as a whole, but its contribution did vary with the intervention being considered. For drugs this was straightforward. The intervention is discrete and there is plenty of good quality research at least in part using the same structured outcome measures (although we have already noted the absence of atypical vs. typical studies). Problems occur where the intervention under consideration can take many complex forms (as in family interventions), making comparison and a subsequent distillation of recommendations complicated. The problem of treatment fidelity brings with it the risk that the effective element of an intervention may get lost in the translation into local practice. This is even more likely when the intervention relies on training that is both scarce and expensive.

The most striking effect of using the EBM approach was the loss of the physical interventions part of our project through lack of any outcome study of effectiveness. Nevertheless, the teams wished to retain it, based partly perhaps on subjective feelings and anecdotal evidence but also in recognition that, at least for cervical screening and mammography, some evidence did exist.

Conclusions

The absence of any accepted treatment guidelines requires clinical effectiveness programmes to develop their own guidelines. It is contentious whether this in itself will make it more likely that those guidelines will be implemented. Furthermore, the chronic and complex nature of schizophrenia poses the risk that guidelines will not be sufficiently focused and so perhaps neither completed nor implemented. The use of an evidence-based medicine approach helped our project avoid this pitfall. By setting narrow clinical questions it was possible to review the relevant literature in a practical and useful way despite the limited resources of the project. However, our lasting impression was that clinical guidelines were most likely to be used by those closely involved in developing them. In mental healthcare, at least, it may be that the way to propagate effective clinical practice is to facilitate the development of guidelines at a local, perhaps even team, level.

6

Referring people with breast problems

GRAHAM HENDERSON

Location

Breast cancer is a particular problem within East Surrey Health Authority, which until recently had one of the highest death rates from this disease in the UK. This is not unexpected, given the relatively affluent nature of the local population, but has nonetheless been a source of concern to both patients and professional groups for some years.

Background

During 1994–95, the then East and Mid Surrey Health Authorities worked closely with professionals from the local trusts, from the Jarvis Breast Screening Unit and with the FHSA to develop the East Surrey Breast Cancer Strategy which, following full agreement between all parties, was formally adopted by the Eastern Surrey Health Commission in April 1995. The strategy set out standards for the services people should expect on referral to hospital or from the breast screening services. These included 'one stop' multi-disciplinary clinics in hospitals, time limits on waiting time for referral to hospital (1 week for urgent cases), waiting time for results and the number of cases a surgeon should see each year to be accepted as a provider of breast services by the commission.

In addition, the strategy recognised that formal guidelines agreed between hospital and primary care services were essential if patients were to be appropriately and expeditiously referred to hospital when necessary, without causing undue anxiety to those individuals who were unlikely to have breast cancer.

As the Breast Cancer Strategy was implemented, a pattern of increasing numbers of referrals, without an increase in the number of breast cancers detected, began to emerge. Information from the breast care teams suggested that this was due to an increased tendency on the part of local GPs to refer patients presenting with breast problems to the rapid-access specialist clinics, in preference to managing them in a primary care setting. Speculation as to the reasons for this included: lack of confidence on the part of GPs in identifying benign breast disease; increased demand from patients for specialist opinion; and a 'supply-led' effect of easy, rapid access to specialists. It was felt that, at least for the first two of these potential causes, education of GPs in the operation of an authoritative, evidence-based guideline would help them to identify appropriate patients for primary care-led management.

If an appropriate guideline could be identified and implemented, therefore, we would expect to see the following improvements in patient care:

- fewer patients in the rapid-access clinics, allowing more consultation time for each

- quicker access to the clinics for those patients needing rapid specialist assessment

- fewer patients referred to hospital who could be treated in primary care, reducing anxiety and time spent in accessing care for the patients.

The guidelines

The guidelines were published by the NHS Breast Screening Programme in late 1995 with a foreword, endorsing them for use by GPs, by the President of the Royal College of General Practitioners. They had been developed by the Breast Screening Programme and the Cancer Research Campaign using an evidence-based consensus approach. A literature review preceded the drafting of the guidelines by a small group, including recognised national authorities. The draft, and then a second draft, were circulated to a number of breast surgeons, and their comments incorporated, and the final version was published under the authorship of the director of the CRC Primary Care Education Research Group, two professors of surgery, a consultant surgeon and a professor of general practice.

Although it was intended that a local referral guideline be produced, production of the national guidelines in the Autumn of 1995 persuaded us that, if they were acceptable locally, we need not produce our own. The guidelines were considered by the local Clinical Protocols Evaluation Committee (a GP-led body) and the local breast consultants, and it was agreed that they could be adopted, unaltered, for local use.

Initially, the guidelines were simply mailed out to each of the 63 local practices but, as will be seen later, this had predictably limited effectiveness. When funding became available, therefore, we were pleased to be able to set up a more sophisticated implementation programme.

Method

Process

We decided to implement the guidelines by undertaking personal visits to each general practice in the East Surrey area. The objective of the visits was to introduce the guidelines to those members of the primary care team who were present; to discuss the operation of the guidelines, answering questions where possible and taking more complex queries away for expert advice; and to distribute copies of the guidelines as required.

Of the 63 practices, 52 (83%) were actually visited during the programme. Only 4 refused the offer of a visit. The visits were usually part of a practice lunchtime meeting, and those present always included some (rarely all) GPs, and often some other members of the team (e.g. practice nurses).

Project supervision

A steering group was set up to advise on the project, and to ensure that a range of views (patients, GPs, etc.) were taken into account. The steering group consisted of:

- members of the two hospital breast care teams
- a GP who we were confident had the confidence of his colleagues (he already had an elected representative role)
- a patient. There proved to be no alternative but to identify a patient from one of the clinics and ask her to participate. We would have preferred to get a nominee from a local patients' representative group, but no such group existed in the district. The patient representative was, however, put in touch with such a group in a neighbouring area for support and advice.

Educational inputs

The primary educational process used was the practice visit described above. It is noteworthy, in the light of the success of the project, that the project worker had neither a primary care nor an educator background. Some educational support was provided for her by the project funding organisation, but the changes in clinical practice that we achieved were essentially accomplished by someone who was neither a trained educator nor a clinician.

As the project progressed it became clear that there were a number of areas in which many GPs had uncertainties about breast disease management, and we decided to supplement the practice visits with two seminars at which GPs could discuss issues directly with the breast care teams.

Audit and monitoring

A substantial proportion of the resources of the project were used in auditing its outcome. First, an initial postal survey of GPs was undertaken to establish whether they could identify all patients presenting over a period of time with breast problems. As only a quarter of respondents were able to do this, it was decided not to undertake the audit of breast disease presenting to general practice which had originally been intended. This questionnaire was also used to find out how many GPs recalled receiving the guidelines from the original mailing, which had occurred some eight months previously. Only half of the responders (20% of all GPs) recalled receiving the guidelines.

The major effort in monitoring the project was committed to performing a pre- and a post-audit of the records of patients attending the rapid-access clinics. All notes and referral letters for all new patients attending at each hospital in three months prior to the project (January–March 1996) and three months after the visits had been completed (March–May 1997) were identified and analysed for appropriateness of the referral. Assessment was done against the criteria set out in the guidelines on a standard proforma, and each referral was classified as 'appropriate' or 'inappropriate'. In addition, the breast consultants completed a separate assessment of appropriateness for each patient in the post-audit period as a validation check.

Results

Preliminary survey

A questionnaire was sent to each GP in the district to test whether they recalled receiving guidelines sent out some eight months earlier (see Table 6.1).

Table 6.1   Results of preliminary questionnaire

Questionnaires sent out	222
Questionnaires returned	89 (40%)
Number of GPs who recalled receiving original mailing of guidelines	44 (50% of responders)

Audit of appropriateness of referrals

A total of 406 GP referrals were made to the two clinics during the pre-audit (January–March 1996), compared with 294 during the post-audit (March–May 1997). However, the number of appropriate referrals dropped by only 16 (6%, not statistically significant), whilst the number of inappropriate referrals (as assessed against the guidelines) dropped by 96 (70%) ($\chi^2 = 34.7$; $p < 0.000001$) (*see* Table 6.2). The change in the proportion of inappropriate referrals was statistically significant for each hospital independently (Unit 1 $\chi^2 = 26.9$; $p < 0.000001$: Unit 2 $\chi^2 = 11.6$; $p = 0.001$).

There was thus a highly significant reduction both in the proportion and the absolute number of inappropriate referrals over the period of the intervention, whilst the number of appropriate referrals remained roughly constant. Total new patient attendances dropped by 28%.

Table 6.2   Changes in inappropriate referrals

	Total referrals		Appropriate referrals		Inappropriate referrals	
	1996	1997	1996	1997	1996	1997
Unit 1	172	133	121	125	51 (30%)	8 (3%)
Unit 2	234	161	147	127	87 (54%)	34 (21%)
Total	**406**	**294**	**268**	**252**	**138** (34%)	**42** (14%)

Further analysis of the referrals shows that the mean age of the appropriate referrals was 48 in the pre-audit period and 49 for the post-audit. The mean age of the inappropriate referrals was 41 before and 40 in the post-audit, suggesting that the two groups come from different populations.

Finally, the number of malignancies diagnosed among these clinic attenders was 30 during the period of the pre-audit and 38 during the post-audit (non-significant change). The results therefore do not suggest that more selective referral was leading to non-referral of patients with malignancies.

Discussion

Achievements

The primary aim of the project was to reduce the number of inappropriate referrals to the rapid-access breast clinics (without reducing the number of appropriate referrals). The results of the audit clearly show that this indeed occurred over the period of the project. Inappropriate referrals were reduced by some 70%, reducing total referrals by 28%, whilst the number of appropriate referrals, and the number of cancers detected, did not change.

Ideally, we would like to show that the educational project *caused* the changes in referral practice. Given that this was an uncontrolled study (there was no control group of GPs who were not offered the intervention), and that cause and effect for behavioural change is usually multi-factorial, definitive proof of effectiveness is not available. However, we should consider some alternative hypotheses for the changes observed.

First, the participants in the study (East Surrey GPs) would have been subject to a range of other influences on their management of breast disease. These include the medical press, mass media and other opportunities for continuing professional development. However, the magnitude of the change, and the observation that referral rates to specialist services tend to rise over time, suggest that these factors are unlikely to have been responsible for the changes observed. There was no other systematic educational effort on this area of practice in the district over the period of the project.

Secondly, it could be suggested that the guidelines themselves, unaccompanied by any other programme, would have brought about the change. Against this is the fact that the guidelines were sent to all GPs two months prior to the period covered by the pre-audit; less than half of the responders to the initial questionnaire recalled receiving them, and the evidence from other research suggests that this approach is generally of limited effectiveness.

Finally, it may be that GPs were simply referring less patients to the clinics for reasons unconnected with the project – long waiting times, for instance. However, this should have resulted in a general reduction in referrals. The results of the audit clearly show that, whilst inappropriate referrals dropped by 70%, appropriate referrals dropped by only 6%, suggesting that whatever had affected referral practice had increased GPs' ability to discriminate between the two types of referral.

We therefore conclude that the project did indeed influence GPs' referral practice in the desired direction, without increasing risk to patients by reducing the number of appropriate referrals.

The objective of reducing inappropriate referrals was, of course, to improve patient care, both by increasing the amount of time available to appropriately referred patients in the clinics, and by enabling people whose problem could be addressed without a hospital referral not to have to go to hospital. No direct measures of gains in these areas are available from the project, but the fact that the number of new patients in the clinics was reduced by 28% means that the opportunity for patients to have more time with the team was made available.

Problems and difficulties

We encountered surprisingly few real problems in carrying out the project, though the following are worth noting.

- One might have expected that lack of local ownership of the guidelines would have affected their acceptability, but this did not prove to be the case on the ground.

- Identifying appropriate patient representation was not easy; as the organiser of one patients' group put it to us 'when you're in treatment, you need to concentrate on getting better, and after that you really want to forget about your illness and get on with your life'. As stated above, we used one of the breast care teams to identify a patient, which worked well in this case but is less than ideal as it may produce a patient who is more satisfied and less critical than the average.

- Making appointments for practice visits was slightly more difficult than anticipated – everyone seemed to prefer Monday lunchtimes – but only 4 out of 63 practices actually refused a visit.

- There were the anticipated problems in finding patient notes, but persistence was rewarded by an eventual 100% tally.

- The two seminars were interesting, but if anything they demonstrated the correctness of the decision not to rely on this approach alone. Attendance was in line with that expected, but inevitably consisted of GPs with a greater than average interest in the field, who are less likely to need professional development in this area than many of their colleagues.

Service implications

One of the central responsibilities of a health authority (HA) is to assess the health needs of its residents, and then to commission services to meet those needs. Increasingly, such services will need to be commissioned in primary care, and will frequently involve changing the existing pattern of clinical practice. This has traditionally been seen as difficult, with many HAs concentrating their efforts to change clinical practice on supporting infrastructure improvements, and relying on the postgraduate education system, over which they have little influence, to address clinical practice. The one consistent exception to this is the network of pharmaceutical advisers attempting to influence prescribing patterns.

The results of this project suggest that it is feasible to bring about changes in clinical practice using non-clinicians as change agents.

Most HAs employ pharmaceutical advisers to visit practices on drug issues; does not the increasing need for guideline-assisted clinical care make the deployment of a 'guideline task force', actively promoting the HA's clinical policies, something that organisations that are serious about a primary care-led NHS should consider?

7

The management of leg ulcers in the community: a multi-disciplinary experience in primary care

ANNMARIE RUSTON AND MIKE LAWES

Location

We describe the multi-disciplinary experience of implementing clinical guidelines for the management of leg ulcers in the community, in the Tunbridge Wells locality of the West Kent Medical Audit Advisory Group. In order to overcome the potential difficulties presented by a variety of contractual arrangements it was decided that the project should be undertaken in fundholding practices which had contracted community nursing services from one provider, Hastings and Rother NHS Trust. Each practice employed its own practice nurses. The consultant staff from the local Kent and Sussex Weald NHS Acute Trust were also consulted.

Background

The care of patients with venous leg ulcers had been a cause of local concern particularly around the boundaries of responsibility between different health professionals. Is the GP personally accountable for the actions of those team members to whom he or she has confidently delegated work? Leg ulcers were recognised as being costly in terms of time and resources, but the potential for improving patient outcomes in relation to healing rates, re-occurrence and quality of life were considered to be great. Adapting nationally formulated guidelines for local use in accordance with the Assisting Clinical Effectiveness Programme was readily accepted in the Tunbridge Wells locality and each GP in the specified practices was invited, by letter, to be involved in the project or to agree to the involvement of their practice.

In order to ensure that the guidelines to be implemented were of a high quality the nationally recommended guidelines on the management of leg ulcers in the community were selected. The overall aim of the project was to facilitate the implementation of locally adapted national guidelines for the management of patients with leg ulcers at the primary care level.

Methods

Based on evidence from the literature it was anticipated that the implementation of clinical guidelines would be expedited more effectively through a pro-active, well-designed programme for the management of the process of change, which included plans and sequences to be performed by the relevant parties and to which all professionals were committed. Therefore, our first task was to set up a 'change management' team to disseminate the guidelines, raise awareness and take responsibility for communication, co-ordination and feedback within their own organisations.

We recognised that effective implementation was likely to be determined by the following factors:

- co-operation and involvement of 'front line' staff or end users of the guidelines

- an understanding of the perspective of patients
- an appropriate educational input
- the availability of time and resources to bring about change.

These criteria were used to determine the composition of the 'change management' team which consisted of district and practice nurses, a nurse manager, a nurse clinical tutor, GPs and patients. The project was conducted through a series of meetings of the team who then fed information and tasks back to their own organisations. Various work groups were set up to carry out individual tasks as necessary. These procedures ensured that all key stakeholders were involved and kept informed of the process throughout the duration of the project.

Dissemination

As part of the initial process of raising awareness of the guidelines, meetings were held with district and practice nurses in their own workplaces. The general practice representative took responsibility for liaising with participating general practitioners, the vascular surgeon, dermatologist and dietician. Participants were asked to consider the national guidelines and to identify potential barriers and facilitating factors, within their professional setting, that might impinge on the successful implementation of the guidelines.

Having raised awareness of the project the next step facing the 'change management' team was to collect the necessary information on which to base the implementation strategy. As any implementation strategy can be seen to affect the structure and/or process of care, it was felt important to identify the potential barriers in terms of these.

Organisational diagnosis

A thorough 'organisational diagnosis' was instigated using four different approaches.

- An examination of administrative, structural and organisational constraints was undertaken through feedback sessions held by team members in their own workplaces.

- A detailed investigation of the context, skills and practices of the nurses was conducted in semi-structured interviews with a sample of nurses. The topics covered included nurses' knowledge, present practice and present methods of updating, training needs and qualification levels.

- The influence of patient behaviour was ascertained via a series of interviews and focus group discussions with patients. The issues covered included patient compliance and satisfaction with the service.

- In order to demonstrate the performance gap between existing practice and 'best practice', as detailed in the guidelines, a retrospective audit was undertaken using a locally adapted version of the Liverpool Audit Tool.

Local adaptation

Duff *et al.* (1996) argue that a potentially important element for the successful implementation of clinical guidelines is a sense of their 'ownership' amongst those carrying out the implementation. We aimed to achieve this through adapting the national guidelines for local use. In order to achieve this a special task group was set up consisting of a GP, a practice nurse, a district nurse, the project facilitator, the local vascular surgeon and the nurse educator. This group used information collected to date, their expertise and local knowledge to adapt the national guidelines to suit local circumstances.

Implementation strategy

Once the locally adapted guidelines were available a strategy development group was appointed to devise the implementation strategy. This group used the evidence collected to devise a four-pronged strategy. Based on feedback from the health professionals involved, the data collected and evidence from the literature it was anticipated that an implementation programme which was designed to fit the needs of nurses and which was an integral part of clinical decision making would stand the greatest chance of success. The resulting strategy was implemented over a three-month period and contained four main elements, documentation, training, supplies and on-going support.

Documentation

The documentation produced to facilitate implementation fell into two categories: documentation essential to decision making and documentation to support the process. A specific wound assessment group was set up to devise an assessment/treatment form to be used by all nurses when treating patients with leg ulcers. The form was designed to lead nurses through an assessment procedure, detail what information was to be recorded and identify suitable treatment regimes. The form was drawn up, in response to feedback from the nurses, to follow the requirements of the locally adapted guidelines. In completing the forms appropriately the nurses would automatically be complying with the guidelines. In addition, nurses were supplied with patient information leaflets to give to patients during the consultation.

Nurses were also supplied with a draft copy of the locally adapted guidelines, a laminated wound assessment card and a graphically illustrated leaflet detailing the key elements of the guidelines.

Training

A comprehensive, flexible training programme was devised and conducted both prior to and during implementation. Prior to implementation a study day covering sessions on the guidelines, pathophysiology, prevention, assessment and management of leg ulcers, and the assessment of pain was provided for nurses. The study day also contained three workshops covering compression bandaging, use of Doppler meters and pain assessment tools. In addition to this the project facilitator provided 'in-house' training in the general practices and in the district nurse base.

During the implementation phase the project facilitator organised six training sessions in the district nurses' base and four in general practices. These training sessions were arranged so that nurses could attend for the whole session or just drop in and stay as long as they needed to cover the areas they felt they were having difficulty with. Additional training was available, on demand, from the project facilitator, and two nurses were designated to cascade information. This was used by those who were unable to leave their workplaces and for patient-specific training.

Supplies

A shortage of Doppler equipment and the fact that the appropriate compression bandaging was not available on FP10 were identified as potential barriers to implementation. Therefore, an essential part of the 'change programme' was the provision of these items.

On-going support

Continual motivation and support was provided by the project facilitator by liaising with all nurses during the implementation stage. This aspect of the programme provided a monitoring of activity and enabled unforeseen factors affecting implementation to be identified.

Monitoring and evaluation

The final tasks to be completed were a repeat audit and evaluation. The audit was conducted after three months and additional information on the use of Dopplers, completion of the forms, use of compression bandaging and healing rates was collected.

The evaluation of the process, from the nurses' perspective, was undertaken by interviewing 20 nurses using a semi-structured schedule. Topics covered included:

- their understanding and the acceptability of the programme
- the effectiveness of the implementation programme
- changes in decision making and treatment of leg ulcers
- factors influencing the adoption of guidelines and
- factors most likely to bring about and sustain a change in clinical practice.

Results

Organisational analysis

The 'organisational analysis' was valuable and enabled us to identify a number of potentially important barriers to implementation. First, all nurses felt that it would be difficult to fit in the time to do an holistic assessment. Secondly, the cost of compression bandaging was problematic. Whilst bandages are prescribable on an FP10, padding is not. Compression bandaging entails greater short-term expense but cost savings in the long term (Morrell *et al.*, 1998). However, some GPs were not prepared to meet the greater expenditure, in the short term, from their existing budgets. A third barrier was a shortage of Dopplers, which made it difficult for practice nurses, in particular, to carry out an accurate assessment of leg ulcers. The fourth difficulty lay in the fact that the information needed to carry out an holistic assessment was not often readily available to practice nurses, thus reducing the quality of the initial assessment. Finally, patient non-compliance was felt to be a considerable potential barrier.

There was a general acceptance of, and positive attitude towards, the aims and objectives of the project amongst the nurses. They felt that the multi-disciplinary nature of the project would facilitate referrals to hospital. However, this enthusiasm was not matched in reality as the interviews with nurses showed that in spite of a good level of knowledge they were not able to put into practice what they knew to be the most appropriate methods of assessment and treatment. In particular, the use of Dopplers was not universal and the measuring and charting of the size of ulcers was not a routine part of practice. Ulcer cleaning techniques varied considerably, as did the number of times a dressing was changed. Very few of the nurses interviewed used any form of pain assessment tool, with the most common forms of pain control being medication, rest and exercise. Finally, although most nurses agreed that preventative health education was vital, only a small proportion provided any for their patients.

The patients' perspective

The main barrier described by patients was pain, this was felt to affect their life-style the most. Dressings that caused offensive smells or were unsightly were also unpopular. Few communication problems were identified; with most nurses being regarded as helpful and informative.

Patients were asked to give their views on the locally adapted guidelines. They felt these were potentially very useful, especially the section covering referral to hospital. However, patients did feel that the type of dressings to be used needed to be individually assessed because of possible reactions to them.

Audits

The audits were conducted pre- and post-implementation and used a 'tool' that consisted of three main sections: nursing assessment, treatment and health education. Each section contained a series of scored activities or criteria, with a total target score at the end of each section. The target score represented 'best practice' and the closer the actual score was to the target score the lower the 'performance gap' was for that particular nurse. The nurses score for each section was arrived at by taking a sample from their caseload and averaging the scores. The data presented in Table 7.1 compare the first and second audit scores for each nurse and shows a general improvement in all scores. In particular, the nursing assessment scores.

Examination of patients' notes also revealed an increase in the number of referrals to the vascular or general surgeon and the

Table 7.1   Comparison of 1st and 2nd audit scores

Audits		Nursing assessment		Treatment		Health		Total education	
Target score		**22**		**11**		**9**		**42**	
		Actual scores							
		1st	2nd	1st	2nd	1st	2nd	1st	2nd
District Nurse	1	12	20	10	11	5	8	27	39
District Nurse	2	14	19	11	9	6	9	31	37
District Nurse	3	18	19	10	11	8	9	36	39
District Nurse	4	15	18	10	11	6	9	31	38
District Nurse	5	9	14	9	10	4	4	22	28
District Nurse	6	12	20	9	10	5	8	26	38
District Nurse	7	17	18	9	11	8	7	34	36
District Nurse	8	15	20	9	11	8	9	32	40
District Nurse	9	15	16	9	10	7	9	31	35
District Nurse 10		20	19	11	11	9	9	40	39
Practice Nurse	1	15	18	11	10	8	8	34	36
Practice Nurse	2	18	19	11	10	9	8	38	37
Practice Nurse	3	14	20	11	11	9	8	34	39
Practice Nurse	4	10	18	10	10	9	9	29	37
Practice Nurse	5	16	17	10	10	9	9	35	36
Practice Nurse	6	17	–	10	–	6	–	33	–

dermatologist. There was also a 50% increase in the number of nurses who were accompanying their patients to hospital to see the consultant. Other improvements included rationalisation of the bandaging and treatments. By the end of the implementation phase compression bandaging was considered for each patient. The majority of the audited notes showed that a Doppler had been used.

Evaluation

Most nurses expressed a positive attitude towards involvement in the project, with the majority seeing it as a means of achieving standardisation in the management of leg ulcers. The perceived benefits of the project were threefold: increased knowledge, skills and confidence, the provision of a more systematic approach to treatment and assessment, and increased communication between health professionals.

The implementation programme was felt to have been comprehensive, meeting the individual needs of most nurses. It was clear that no one particular part of the programme would have been sufficient to meet the needs of all nurses. The district nurses identified three factors constituting the most effective elements of the programme from their perspective. These were the provision of Doppler equipment, individual training provided by the project facilitator and the presence of the project facilitator. The practice nurses, on the other hand, almost unanimously felt that the project facilitator provided the greatest contribution to the success of the programme.

A critical measure of the effectiveness of the implementation programme was the extent to which a change in practice had occurred. Nurses were found to fall into three categories: those whose decision making and treatment had changed substantially, those whose decision making and treatment had become more systematic and those who had not changed their practice. Only seven of the 20 nurses said that they had implemented the full recommendations of the guidelines: six had implemented the assessment aspects and four the treatment aspects of the guidelines. The remainder considered that they were already working in accordance with the guidelines.

Conclusions

Clinical effectiveness is a central feature of NHS policy. However, its implementation is a complex process involving three main stages: first, providing information or evidence of effectiveness of specific healthcare interventions; secondly, bringing about change in practice through education, clinical guidelines and audit; and thirdly, monitoring progress. The project described in this chapter was concerned essentially with the second and third stages, bringing about change and monitoring progress. The evidence of effectiveness utilised in this study was derived from the NHSE recommended guidelines for the management of leg ulcers in the community; they were, however, locally adapted.

The 'Management of leg ulcers in the community' project was relatively successful in facilitating this complex process and there were a number of key features that can be seen to have contributed to it meeting its aims and objectives.

1 The project used existing 'knowledge' or evidence from the literature to identify relevant 'management of change' theories and successful implementation strategies. This information was synthesised and then used to underpin the overall design of the project. However, the implementation strategy was subject to continual formative evaluation by participants and was adapted as necessary.

2 A second essential element of the project was the thorough analysis of the current situation. As any implementation strategy can be seen to affect the structure and/or process of care, it was important to determine potential barriers to implementation in these terms. A pre-condition to successful change requires a detailed understanding of the context into which the change is introduced and a current 'organisational diagnosis'.

3 The establishment of an acceptable, effective and committed 'management of change' team was an essential feature of the success of the project. The team included district and practice nurses, representatives from nursing education, management, GPs and patients. Even more important than the constitution of the management team itself was the appointment of a locally known and respected district nurse as the project facilitator. This appointment ensured that the dissemination of the guidelines and the introduction of the project to participants was carried out with an understanding of the language, context and problems of the staff who were being asked to take part.

4 Although the project used nationally commended guidelines, it was recognised that one of the central issues in the development and implementation of guidelines is that of 'ownership', or acceptance by those who have responsibility for using them. Involving nurses in the local adaptation of the guidelines helped to ensure their needs were met and made the changes seem less threatening.

5 Success depended on the development and implementation of effective strategies to bring about change. Based on evidence collected as part of the organisational diagnosis it was decided that a strategy that was an integral part of the clinical consultation and decision making would stand the greatest chance of success.

6 Tight project management and adherence to project milestones were essential to ensure that the project did not lose momentum.

The success of this project depended on the satisfactory interaction of a number factors and it would have been unrealistic to underestimate the problems encountered. For example, the time-scale of the project was very tight and it was felt that a three-month implementation period was very short to see the full benefits for patients.

The treatment/assessment form devised as part of the implementation strategy was criticised by nurses because of the time required for completion. However, those nurses who had the most leg ulcer patients during the implementation phase gained speed through practice in completing the form. The majority of nurses valued the form because it meant that they did not have to rely on their memory to collect the information needed, they were able to be more systematic.

Another problem that needed to be overcome was dealing with the competing demands of ensuring the evidence base of the guidelines was maintained and at the same time incorporating the views or practices of local specialists. For example, after consultation with the vascular surgeon, consideration of referral for vascular reconstruction in order to reduce recurrence was included in the guidelines; however, the evidence base for the value of surgery in preventing recurrence is limited and conflicting.

Nevertheless, the project achieved an overall improvement in the assessment and treatment of leg ulcers, increased communication levels between practitioners and achieved a positive health gain for patients.

Since the completion of the project the use of the locally adapted guidelines has been extended to include the other local community trust. The facilitator who worked on the project has also been asked to introduce the guidelines to the local NHS Acute Trust staff.

The results of this study have provided good evidence which can be used to inform future commissioning decisions. West Kent Health Authority has been very supportive and, clearly, decisions will need to be made about the future funding of compression bandaging and Doppler machines by the health authority and NHS trusts.

8

The management of leg ulcers in the Merton and Sutton Community NHS Trust

CERIE NICHOLAS

Location

In June 1991, 18 district nurses and one locality nurse manager in the community trust covering Merton and Sutton Health Authority formed a network of satellite nurses with the aim of improving care services for patients who had leg ulcers. They served approximately 332 900 people, coming from a variety of ethnic and socio-economic backgrounds in south-west London.

Background

Leg ulcers are a common problem, estimated to cost the NHS between £294 000 000 and £650 000 000 per year. Complete healing of leg ulcers can take years and recurrence is a problem. Most care is provided by community nurses but, despite considerable research, the exact methods of treatment remain controversial (Effective Health Care No. 4, 1997). Recent research has confirmed that a community-based leg ulcer clinic, with trained nurses, using Doppler and bandaging is more effective than traditional home-based treatment (Morrell *et al.*, 1998).

The aim of the project was to reduce ulcer healing times and prevent ulcer recurrence incidence through the implementation of national guidelines on managing leg ulcers. Through this approach, all nurses should be proficient in the treatment of leg ulcers and provide expert advice to patients. To achieve this a number of separate areas of activity were envisaged (*see* Box 8.1).

Box 8.1

1   To review and establish service needs within each locality

2   To produce local baseline information on practice before and after implementation of guideline

3   To work closely with GPs and practice nurses to provide continuity of treatment and care

4   To establish working relationships with hospital doctors and nurses in the area

5   To set up staff support networks

6   To involve the patients within the leg ulcer clinics on this project to define potential problems within the guidelines and action plans, and to adopt these before implementation takes place

7   To prevent the recurrence of leg ulcers through health education and promotion

Situation prior to the project

- We had written a Standard of Care.

- Each nurses' base had purchased a Doppler machine and Polaroid camera.

- Basic training had been given to satellite nurses to establish local updating within their nursing teams. They also maintained an up-date resource folder.

- Talks had been given to GPs.

- We had produced a health promotion leaflet on leg ulcer care.

- We had opened nine leg ulcer clinics across the district.

We felt we were starting from a strong position and Box 8.2 shows a summary of the workload in 1995.

Box 8.2 Leg ulcer report 1995		
Total number of patients:		**2100**
1993–94	2097	
1992–93	1330	
Increase of contacts:		**3**
Time in hours:		**19 491**
1993–94	19 620	
1992–93	17 933	
Decrease of hours:		**159**
Number of contacts:		**35 129**
Compared with 1993–94	35 378	
Compared with 1992–93	32 803	
Decrease of contacts:		**249**
Average face-to-face contact:		**33 minutes**

There was not, however, the facility to monitor the specific outcome of leg ulcer care in the information system functioning at that time.

Method

Appointing a project co-ordinator

To enable implementation of the guidelines to take place we envisaged one person taking a lead and linking with satellite nurses to develop action plans for improvements. The post holder would:

- translate the national guidelines into locally accepted guidelines
- co-ordinate the link between hospital and community
- develop training packages for satellite nurses to cascade information to other members of the nursing team
- co-ordinate the audit of leg ulcers both before and after implementation
- identify a users group to assist with the implementation of this project
- work closely with hospital vascular surgeons, dermatologists and nurses, and participate in the leg ulcer clinics in the hospitals
- work with the satellite nurses in each base
- link with the practice nurses and GPs in GP surgeries
- keep the purchasers informed of the progress of the project through the quality department.

A timetable was drawn up

A leg ulcer facilitator was put in post in July 1996 to implement the project.

	Time plan
1 Appointment of leg ulcer facilitator to co-ordinate and establish joint working practices between hospital and community.	May 1996
2 Develop a user focus group to assist in the project.	June 1996
3 To look at the new guidelines and develop our current standards in line with these.	July 1996
4 To carry out an audit of leg ulcer management building upon the recent work.	July 1996
5 To develop a training programme to support the evidence, which can be cascaded to other members of nursing team through satellite nurses.	September 1996
6 To implement the local leg ulcer guidelines.	December 1996
7 Re-audit leg ulcer management to compare with first audit to identify improvements made and further work to be done.	March 1997

Obtaining user views (GPs, district nurses, patients)

A user focus group was envisaged but found not to be suitable because:

- GPs did not feel they wished to participate in such a group
- patients, because of age and poor mobility, felt it was difficult to attend a group meeting.

It was decided to conduct in-depth semi-structured interviews instead. Twenty-two patients, four GPs and four practice nurses from all areas of the trust were interviewed.

Follow-up letters and information have been sent to all concerned.

Undertaking clinical audit

An assessment on the healing time of venous leg ulcers was completed just before the start of the project. The objective of this audit was to look at the healing of leg ulcers over a period of 16 weeks and to see whether the size of the ulcers reduced over this period. The audit was carried out at all leg ulcer clinics in September 1996. First, we looked at the date of the first examination and last examination and calculated the number of weeks over which treatment took place, the size of the leg ulcer before and after treatment, which resulted in a total healing area and average healing area per week, and, finally, whether a compression bandage was used.

The intention was to repeat the assessment at the completion of the project, but we felt that we should gain far more information than a simple measurement of ulcer size. In view of this and the availability of new technology, we devised a new follow-up assessment which commenced 1 January 1997 and was completed by June 1997. As well as healing rates this gave us information on nutrition levels, pain management, compliance, referrals and the cost of healing in time and materials. This provided valuable data for further studies

A new assessment form for leg ulcers was devised, based on these guidelines, which reduced the amount of writing, encouraged a *full* assessment and, by its format, made diagnosis more obvious. This was evaluated in a pilot study and is now used by all community nurses in the trust.

Choosing guidelines

Nationally recognised guidelines and those of other trusts were collected and reviewed. Our existing practice was already close to the guidelines produced by the NHS Executive Consensus Strategy, Liverpool 1997, and did not require too much revision, but some aspects (e.g. monitoring pain levels and follow-up of healed ulcers) had not previously been emphasised. Following the project, the *Effective Health Care Bulletin* on compression therapy for venous leg ulcers was published. The Royal College of Nursing is creating guidelines based on this review, which were to be published in late 1998.

In addition, a dressing protocol was written, printed and distributed to all trained staff, in response to their request for clarification on the use of various wound care products. Following this, the pharmaceutical advisers for Merton, Sutton and Wandsworth HA and the Merton and Sutton Community NHS Trust invited me to write a section on wound care products which was included in the District Formulary.

Implementation

In order to implement the guidelines, it was necessary to inform all staff of their importance. The Wound Care Satellite Group's enthusiasm helped us to cascade this to their bases. Visits to nurses' bases and leg ulcer clinics and discussion groups reinforced the message and a copy of the guidelines was distributed to every trained nurse in the trust.

Assessing the district nurses' knowledge of the management of leg ulcers

The Liverpool Audit Tool was used for this purpose as it has been well tested and reflects the principles of the national guidelines and our own. It was felt to be important that the nurses' knowledge be measured against external standards of research-based 'best practice'. This was considered to be less threatening and a realistic goal for all nurses.

There are several ways of using this tool but an interview schedule was chosen as being the most appropriate.

Results

Interviews with four general practitioners

Questions asked were as follows.

What happens when a patient with a leg ulcer comes to you?

Do you give any information on medical history etc. to the nurses?

When do you think it necessary to refer a leg ulcer patient?

How does the type of leg ulcer influence your referral?

How do you decide on the treatment for leg ulcers?

What is your response when a district nurse feels that investigations or referral to a consultant is required?

What feedback do you receive from the district nurses?

What other feedback would you like to receive?

In general there was considerable variation in the responses, depending on the GPs' perceptions of their knowledge and the capacity of their practice nurse to cope. However, most considered that the main responsibility for ulcers was with the nurses and allowed them to refer on if they considered it necessary.

Interviews with four practice nurses

Questions asked were as follows.

What happens when a patient with a leg ulcer comes to you?

What information to you provide about the patients? Is a medical history given routinely?

When do you think it necessary to refer?

How does the type of ulcer influence your referral?

How do you decide on treatment for leg ulcers?

What past training have you received on leg ulcers?

What future training on leg ulcer management would you like?

*What suggestions would you make to improve the district nursing leg
ulcer service?*

The role of the leg ulcer facilitator was welcomed and practice
nurses hoped to be able to use her as a resource. The practice
nurses who worked at the same bases as the district nurses referred
directly to them and it appeared that liaison was effective. Practice
nurses who did not work from the same premises gave the responsibility of contact to the patients. This also appeared to be effective
and enabled an appointment to be made by the patient. The district
nurse used this opportunity to request the patient to bring their
medication and a urine specimen with them at the first visit.

It appeared that very little or no information was given to the
nurses at the leg ulcer clinic. Two practice nurses gave no information at all and said the district nurses would elicit any information
from the patient. One listed the types of dressings that had been
tried in the past and one just said that healing was a problem.
Three nurses waited for several weeks or months before referring a
non-healing ulcer. One would refer if the ulcer was very large or
taking months to heal. It might be appropriate to give guidelines
on what information is required by the district nurse clinic and
how soon to refer. A referral form for practice nurses and GPs has
been devised, which may overcome these problems, but further
training is needed in recognising stages of healing and choice of
dressings.

None of the practice nurses had access to a Doppler and none felt
they could determine the aetiology of an ulcer. Three said they
would, therefore, refer all non-healing ulcers. One nurse (25%)
would refer large or persistent ulcers.

The lack of training and equipment gives cause for concern. As
the treatment for venous and arterial ulcers is different and the
consequences of wrong treatment so drastic, it is essential that a
correct assessment of the ulcer is made.

On further questioning, the practice nurses said they realised that
putting compression on an ischaemic leg could cause damage so
they did not apply compression very often. Since the cornerstone of

treatment of venous ulcers is compression, this indicated that many patients were not getting effective treatment. This emphasises the need for further training and provision of equipment.

When deciding a treatment for leg ulcers it became apparent that choice of dressing was the only consideration. None of them discussed diet, smoking or life-styles with patients. They did not encourage specific exercises, apply compression or measure for stockings. Blood pressure and urinalysis were not usually recorded. Again, this indicates a need for training.

As practice nurses are not part of the community trust, they do not always have the same training opportunities. They are actually invited to attend some of the wound care update sessions held by the trust and some are able to take advantage of these. It may be beneficial if some joint clinics were set up so that expertise could be shared. In some parts of the borough practice nurses are beginning to hold their own leg ulcer clinics. Some have a district nurse quali-fication and feel quite competent but others are looking to gain training in this field. This may be an opportunity for education. Some method needs to be found for different disciplines to exchange skills and knowledge to their mutual benefit and improved service to the patients.

Results of patient interviews

In view of the generalisability of this information the results are presented in more detail.

Questions asked were as follows.

1 *How were you referred to the leg ulcer clinic?*

2 *How long did you have your ulcer before asking for help?*

3 *What did the district nurse discuss with you when you first attended?*

4 *What problems do you have with your leg ulcer?*

5 *How did the nurse deal with these problems?*

6 *What information did the nurse give you on the following – exercise, diet, smoking?*

7 *What changes can you see in your leg ulcer?*

8 *What information has the nurse given you about preventing the ulcer from recurring?*

9 *How would you improve the service?*

The responses were as follows.

1 The majority of patients [14 (64%)] were referred to the clinic by their GP. Three (14%) had been visited at home by district nurses then referred when they became more mobile. Three (14%) were referred by the hospital when they discontinued their clinic. Two (9%) were self-referrals. These two patients had had previous ulcers and were aware of the existence of the clinics.

2 Twelve patients (55%) had an ulcer for less than 4 weeks before seeking help, four (18%) for 1–3 months, one (5%) for under 6 months, two (9%) for almost a year and three (14%) for over one year. Those waiting for over 6 months before visiting a profes-sional had a long history of recurrent ulceration (35 years, 20 years and 3–4 years) and thought they could treat it themselves. They sought help when no progress was made.

3 It was significant that 11 patients (50%) could not remember anything about their first attendance regarding advice, examina-tion or explanation. Eight per cent of these patients were over 75 years. Seventy per cent had had ulcers for more than a year, and it was not possible to determine if this high incidence was due to memory problems, perception difficulty or inability of nurses to communicate effectively. Further study needs to be made to facil-itate health education. Six patients (27%) recalled physical exami-nation and tests. Two patients (9%) remembered advice and compression. As compression is the cornerstone of treatment for venous leg ulcers, this seems a low figure and could explain the problems with compliance sometimes found. Only three patients (14%) said they received an information leaflet although it is standard practice to give one to each new patient. Further inves-tigation is needed to determine if the first visit is the appropriate time to give this, or how many nurses go through the leaflet

with the patient? Will they read it? Can they read it? Does it need reinforcement – if so when? Constraints of time are a problem, but a way must be found to inform and collaborate with patients.

4 Pain appeared to be the main problem for patients with an ulcer. This bears out recent research which states that, contrary to previous thinking, patients with *venous* ulcers experience considerable pain. Twelve patients (55%) declared that pain was a problem. Infection was a factor for three patients (14%), leakage of dressings for three (14%), eczema was a problem for two (9%) patients and one patient (5%) had reduced mobility: this was surprisingly low but perhaps the age of the majority of patients (over 65) affected their expectation of mobility.

   1 – (5%) disliked stockings

   1 – (5%) declared he was unable to swim

   5 – (23%) said their ulcers caused them no problems

   12 – (55%) said that the nurse had dealt with their problems

   5 – (23%) had no problems. The ulcer did not affect their lifestyle.

5 Most patients found that the nurses suggested remedies for their problems. All infections were dealt with by referring to the GP for antibiotics. Eczema was treated topically. When possible, the type of dressing was changed if leakage became a problem. One patient felt he needed to attend clinic twice a week for this. The majority of untreated problems were related to pain control. Some patients did not feel that they needed to involve the nurse and took analgesia when required, others would have liked suggestions of other strategies for pain relief. Pain control will be in the new guidelines and checked at each visit using a visual analogue scale.

6 The results of questions on exercise, diet and smoking gave rise to some concern. On exercise, 11 patients (50%) said they had been given information but 11 (50%) said they had not. On diet

eight patients (36%) said they received information on diet. Ten patients (45%) remembered smoking being discussed.

On further questioning, many patients assumed that diet referred to their weight and many felt defensive about it if they were overweight. This may have had an effect on their memory of the question. Perhaps an equal emphasis on protein, vitamin and mineral intake would reduce a 'block' of memory. 'Smoking' may have produced a similar effect although many who said they cannot remember being asked about it are non-smokers so it may have seemed irrelevant.

7 When asked what changes they could see in their leg ulcer since attending the clinic, 22 (100%) said that there was an improvement. This was especially pleasing in the patients who had ulcers of long duration, as these are most difficult to heal.

8 When asked what information they had received about preventing further ulceration three patients (14%) mentioned protection support and skin care, one (5%) remembered support, one (5%) recalled exercise and elevation, seven (32%) said they had had no information at all and five (23%) said that their ulcers had not healed yet – a valid point. Perhaps the question might be altered to indicate that further ulceration is possible even before a previous ulcer is healed.

In some clinics patients are followed up monthly to ensure compliance with stockings, skin care, diet and exercise, but other clinics feel they are overpressed already. The new guidelines will recommend that patients are checked and re-Dopplered every three months after healing. An argument could be made that this is more cost effective than dealing with a new open ulcer but staff levels may not permit it.

9 Suggestions for improving the leg ulcer clinic service were varied. Fifteen patients (68%) said they felt no improvements were required and that they were very satisfied. Comments ranged from 'good' to 'wonderful' and all praised the attitudes of the nurses. Four patients (18%) thought that the nurses were very busy and that more staff were required; one (5%) felt that he did not want to bother the busy nurses with questions. In a

bustling clinic the nurses have to give the impression that questions are welcome. Would a 'question card' filled in before clinic and handed to the nurse alert her to this problem?

One patient (5%) emphasised that seeing the same nurse each time gave better continuity of care.

Two patients (9%) stated their preference for experienced nurses (sisters) because they appeared more skilled. With increased responsibilities, other grades of staff will help run clinics, most of them are well trained in wound care. Emphasis must be on training less experienced staff in order to maintain standards.

One patient (5%) requested twice weekly clinics. Two clinics do hold two sessions and find it beneficial, but others have staff and room problems which prevent them from providing a second session.

Three patients (14%) felt that they would like more information and advice. When prompted they were unsure of what they required but would like time to express their concerns about their ulcer. One (5%) of these patients thought that a consultant surgeon would be reassuring to have on the premises. Would a visit to her GP give enough reassurance?

Two patients (9%) commented on the difficulties encountered obtaining prescribed dressings. This entailed a visit to the GP to request a prescription, a second visit to obtain it, a visit to the chemist and often a heavy bag to carry to the clinic. Some clinics have no space to store items and this can be a problem. Other clinics have solved this by the GP faxing the chemist and delivery of the items to the clinic or for the nurse to collect. It would be useful to explore other options.

One patient (5%) requested an appointment system which he felt would be fairer. Most clinics do have one that works well. At his clinic transport is provided by an Age Concern minibus so 6–8 patients arrive at once. It would be difficult to implement an appointment system in this case – perhaps negotiation between patients could solve the problem.

Two other patients (9%) said that waiting times are much reduced. No waiting would be ideal and is achieved by some clinics but as patients with problems are seen without an appointment, this can affect the timetable.

Three patients (14%) felt that the service should be more widely publicised. Until referred they did not know about it. When being first set up, posters advertising the clinics were put in surgeries, chemists, supermarkets and community centres. This generated some interest at the time. Perhaps we should confer with Health Education to advertise clinics more widely. This may have an impact on the required staffing levels.

One patient (5%) found wheelchair access was difficult and also required a rail to assist balance near the doors. Access for people with a disability is being addressed at health premises and it is hoped to respond to this problem.

In one clinic a patient (5%) felt that tea facilities would be a good idea. He has been asked for ideas to implement this.

The most notable and disturbing finding has been the high number of patients who say they have not received any health education or discussion of the causes and prevention of leg ulceration. The high recurrence rate of venous ulceration makes it a lifelong problem and patients need clear information so that they can work in partnership with nurses and participate in their treatment on an equal, responsible level. Patient-focused care must not be just a phase. Nurses must encourage patients to ask questions until they understand the best way to manage their disease. In this way compliance will be improved, collaboration will be realistic and clinical effectiveness will be achieved.

First audit, 1995

The minimum number of weeks for treatment was two and the maximum was 36, which gave an average of 10.42 weeks for treatment to take place and the wound to heal.

It can be seen from Table 8.1 that most people had their leg ulcers between 1 and 4 weeks before district nurses became involved in their treatment. Table 8.2 shows the total area before and after treatment and the percentage of area that has healed.

From Table 8.2 it can be seen that 13 out of 20 clients had ulcers

Table 8.1   Length of time with leg ulcer before being seen by district nurse

Straight away	5	(20.8%)
Less than 1 week	4	(16.7%)
1 to 4 weeks	7	(29.1%)
1 to 2 months	1	(4.2%)
2 to 4 months	3	(12.5%)
4 to 6 months	0	
More than 6 months	4	(16.7%)

totally healed within the time of the audit. In addition the average amount of healing was 1.67 cm per week; 84% used compression bandages.

Nurses' knowledge prior to implementation of guidelines

Fifty-two district nurses who were most involved with leg ulcer management were interviewed prior to the implementation of the guidelines. The interviews covered a variety of areas.

1 Nursing assessment of patients with leg ulcers.

2 Nursing treatment of patients with leg ulcers.

3 Health advice and education.

4 General factors.

5 Totals.

Thirty-nine district nurses (75%) achieved 80% or more (which was judged to be the acceptable level) and 13 district nurses (25%) did not achieve 80% These 25% were re-audited at the end of the project.

High marks were achieved by most nurses on health education, 45 (87%), and general factors, 41 (79%). Thirty-three (63%) were

Table 8.2 Areas of leg ulcers before and after treatment

Total area before treatment (cm)	Total area after treatment (cm)	Total area healed (cm)	% of area healed
9	0.25	8.75	97.2
0.04	0	0.04	100
8.75	0	8.75	100
0.25	0	0.25	100
0.25	0	0.25	100
0.5	0	0.5	100
10.5	0.25	10.25	97.6
3	0	3	100
0.125	0	0.125	100
24.5	4	20.5	83.6
2.5	2.5	0	0
4	0	4	100
126	0	126	100
16	0	16	100
75	48	27	36
4	1.5	2.5	62.5
2	0.125	1.875	93.75
2	0	2	100
4	0	4	100

good at assessment and 34 (65%) achieved good marks for treatment.

Using the results of the audit, deficits were identified and training packages developed to remedy them.

Nurses achieving less than 80% overall were re-audited at the end of the project. Of these 13, only two failed to achieve 80%, two were unable to present themselves for re-audit and the remainder had improved scores. Some admitted that they had been disappointed in their previous marks and were determined to use the training programme to improve their performance. Others said that they knew that they would have a repeat audit and updated themselves accordingly. Either way, it was an encouraging response. Several nurses felt more confident after gaining a high score and wished to further their knowledge, requesting topics for inclusion in the programme.

Re-audit, January – June 1997

Thirty-three patients were assessed and detailed information was obtained on referral patterns, history of previous ulcer, use of Doppler, mobility, nutritional status, pain level, type and time of assessment, size and healing times.

Size

The area of ulcers varied from 0.3^2 to 62.7^2. The average size was 4 cm^2, which was the same as for the previous audit.

Healing times

Out of 33 patients, 17 (52%) had fully healed, compared with 70% in the previous audit. The average healing time for these ulcers was 4 weeks, compared with 8 weeks in the previous audit.

Conclusions

This project raised the profile of leg ulcer management both within and outside the trust. The guidelines have been incorporated into the assessment forms used by all nursing staff and have improved the standard of care. An on-going programme of nurse education in wound care has been developed and multi-disciplinary education has been extended.

9

Managing acute, severe asthma

MADELEINE ST CLAIR

Location

This project implemented the British Thoracic Society (1993) guide-lines in an acute hospital setting. The Mid Sussex NHS Trust is an integrated trust offering a full range of acute and community services. Initiatives to improve the quality of clinical care are supported and managed by the trust's Clinical Effectiveness Department staffed by 1.5 whole-time equivalent posts.

Background

Asthma is the commonest chronic disease affecting all age groups in the UK. It is a major cause of preventable death and ill health. The prevalence of asthma is difficult to measure, but it is estimated that in the UK up to 13% of children and about 8% of adults are affected (Anderson *et al.*, 1994). The effective management of asthma is a high priority for patients, purchasers and primary and acute services.

There are well-established guidelines for the management of asthma in several circumstances. The British Thoracic Society (BTS) Asthma Guidelines target five key areas:

1 management of chronic asthma in adults

2 management of chronic asthma in children

3 acute severe asthma in adults

4 acute severe asthma in children

5 acute severe asthma in adults in general practice.

The Mid Sussex NHS Trust project focused on the implementation of the guidelines for acute severe asthma in hospital only.

At the beginning of 1996 the trust established an Asthma Guidelines Steering Group which determined to develop an Integrated Care Pathway (ICP) for the condition. This allowed for the formal integration of asthma care guidelines into daily in-patient care, ensuring educational input and discharge planning arrangements.

However, this was just one part of the Mid Sussex Asthma Management initiative. It was envisaged that there would be further developments to promote community asthma education, including a patient education centre, open access services and a helpline.

Funding was obtained from the ACE programme for the appointment of a Respiratory Nurse Specialist (three days a week) to co-ordinate the development, implementation and evaluation of the ICP and the programme for education. The project was managed by the steering group and endorsed by our key purchasers, and the trust chief executive.

Method

Baseline analysis

Prior to the project a review of asthma services within the trust was undertaken and revealed several points (*see* Table 9.1).

Table 9.1   Results of the review of asthma services

Positive points	Opportunities for improvement
• The medical staff at the trust had knowledge of relevant asthma care guidelines. • The physical and pharmacological care for patients with asthma was of a high standard. • The nursing staff on the medical wards were well trained in the skills of asthma care and monitoring. • There was appropriate equipment (oximeters, peak flow meters) available in all areas which care for patients with acute severe asthma.	• Patients' education/ information about their asthma, self-management and discharge planning was incomplete. • The nursing staff were often too busy to spend time on patient education and check inhaler technique. • Follow-up arrangements and links with primary care were weak. • Nursing staff on non-medical wards were not well trained in the skills of asthma care and monitoring.

There were a number of antecedent conditions in favour of implementing the BTS guidelines and using an ICP, including:

• management of asthma was a priority for patients, the trust, GPs and our purchasers

• the existence of robust guidelines

• the recent appointment of a chest physician with experience in developing ICPs

• the existence of a part-time clinical nurse specialist trained in asthma management.

Aims and objectives

The overall aim was to provide a well-organised, comprehensive service for adults with acute severe asthma, that promoted best practice, was evidence based and accorded with the British Thoracic Society (BTS) guidelines.

Objectives for the project were identified under three main headings.

1 *Educational objectives*

    (i) To extend knowledge and skills on the management of patients with asthma to all healthcare professionals.

    (ii) To promote self-management in order to reduce acute attendances and readmissions.

    (iii) To ensure agreed management of this condition between primary and secondary services.

2 *Organisational objectives*

    (i) To develop an evidence-based integrated care pathway which ensures a unified approach for the care of adults with asthma that is multi-professional, collaborative and uses resources most appropriately.

    (ii) To ensure this approach is recognised and accepted across acute and primary care services.

    (iii) To ensure that individuals with difficult or acute problems have access to education as well as specialist services.

3 *Communication objectives*

    (i) To improve the continuity of care by discharge planning.

Developing standards of care

The BTS guidelines and our own survey of current literature on standards of care were incorporated into the integrated care pathway. Meetings separate from the steering group were established for writing the pathway. Each professional group was responsible for their part.

The ICP was to replace other forms of documentation, including nursing care plans. This would be from the time of admission to the A&E department to the time of transfer back to the GP and home.

Collaboration

Working partnerships and lines of communication were agreed at the beginning of the project. To achieve this we ensured that key stakeholders contributed to the construction of the ICP and to monitoring. We used a 'collaboration by doing' approach and regular feedback.

Patient (user) involvement

Both a user and a representative from the National Asthma Campaign were involved in the steering group, the education of staff, the evaluation of the project and in the presentation of results to hospital staff.

Educational support

Educational support for staff included workshops, ward-based seminars, doctors' sessions and one-on-one sessions. A mixture of users and the multi-professional team (MPT) taught all sessions.
    Opportunities for professional development included:

- special days on care of patients with asthma for staff

- English National Board (ENB) 998 and ICP facilitators course for the Clinical Nurse Specialist (CNS)

- ENB-accredited course on asthma for two members of the medical ward nursing staff.

Monitoring

Project plan. The steering group monitored the project plan and the activity of the CNS (*see* Table 9.3 on pp 102–4).

Use of the ICP. Use of the ICP document in preference to other documentation was calculated by comparing the names and number of adults admitted with acute severe asthma with the number of completed ICPs for these same individuals during the study period.

Standards of care. A retrospective audit of the quality of patient care given was undertaken on all adults (over the age of 18 years) admitted to the trust between August 1996 and February 1997 with a primary diagnosis of acute severe asthma. Audit indica-

Table 9.2 Audit indicators

Aspect of care	Indicator	Standard set by trust
1 Assessment on admission	a Peak expiratory flow (PEF) is to be recorded on admission.	100%
	b If oxygen saturation is below 92% arterial blood gases should be taken.	100%
	c Systemic steroids should be administered on admission.	100%
2 Management in hospital	a 24 hours before discharge the highest and lowest PEF should be recorded and the variability calculated. Discharge from hospital needs to be delayed if the % variability is greater than 25%.	100%
3 Discharge from hospital	a All patients should be discharged on inhaled steroids.	100%
	b All patients should be given an out-patient appointment.	100%
	c All patients should be given a written self-management plan.	100%
	d All patients should be advised to see their GP within 1 week of discharge.	100%

tors were adopted from the BTS minimum data set for standards of care developed by Fazakerley Hospital (*see* Table 9.2). Information against these key indicators was collected by the CNS from both the ICP and patient notes and care plans.

User satisfaction with information received. A survey of users' satisfaction with information received about their asthma during their stay in hospital was undertaken. This was with adults attending a one-week follow-up out-patient appointment with the CNS during February. Information was collected using adapted versions of two questionnaires, the 'illness perception questionnaire' and the 'beliefs about medicines questionnaire'. Adaptation of the questionnaires was undertaken in collaboration with Dr R Horne of the University of Brighton.

Users were asked to complete the questionnaires before their appointment with the CNS. Users completed a further, third, questionnaire covering what they understood about their asthma. These questions were derived from the key areas of information the CNS had discussed with users during their hospital stay.

Statistical analysis

For the BTS minimum data set, differences between the frequency of response between the 1995 national audit and the 1997 trust data are reported using chi square. Fisher's exact probability is also reported where one of the expected cell frequencies was less than 5.0.

Results

Project plan. Overall, the project met its main objectives and completed key stages of the programme within the one-year timeframe and within budget. This included the development and implementation of the ICP and provision of education to staff and carers (*see* Table 9.3).

Table 9.3 Project plan

Date*	Activity	Comments
April 1996 *April 1996*	Briefing day	
May 1996 *May 1996*	Appoint Clinical Nurse Specialist (CNS)	• CNS in post
May 1996 *May 1996*	Steering Group review project	• Lit. review for BTS Guidelines • ICP project team/date • Education project team/ programme/date • Steering Group dates
May 1996 *May 1996*	Commence ICP development concurrent with education	• Set dates • Invitations/venue • Education planned. 1998 for CNS
July 1996 *July 1996*	Pilot ICP on medical wards	• 24 July pilot for two months. Green folders • A&E dept initiative • Staff education. Ward-based sessions and doctors sessions. Multi-professional involvement. Workshops planned • Posters for peak flows • Patient education. Hospital admissions only. Handouts, leaflets and booklets
July 1996 *August 1996*	Network day	• CNS and Manager, Clinical Effectiveness Department

Table 9.3 *continued*

Date*	Activity	Comments
July 1996 *August 1996*	Steering Group	• Reviewed progress. Audit topics finalised
Sept 1996 *Sept 1996*	Finalise pathway and education programme Training on ICPs to other clinical areas	• Minor changes to ICP, otherwise accepted • Roll out to other wards launched by two workshops 12–13 September – 60 delegates • Ward-based education and doctor education to continue • Local GP interest
Oct 1996 *Oct 1996*	Introduce ICP to other clinical areas	• Initial feedback positive. ICP great help with medical outliers • National Asthma Week
Oct 1996 *Dec 1996*	Network day	• Consultant physician
Nov 1996 *Oct 1996*	Steering Group	• Feedback from network day • Feedback from workshops • Results of launch • Project plan review
Jan 1997 *Jan 1997*	Audit projects commence	• BTS standards of care minimum data set • Users satisfaction with information received • The use of the ICP

Table 9.3   *continued*

Date*	Activity	Comments
March 1997 *March 1997*	Steering Group	• Friday, 21 March, Downsmere
April 1997 *April 1997*	Network day	• Wednesday, 23 April, St George's

*Target date, with date achieved in italics.

Use of the ICP. Between 12 August 1996 and 2 February 1997, 33 patients with the primary diagnosis of acute severe asthma were admitted to the trust. Of these, 29 were admitted directly to one of the two acute medical wards, two were admitted to a general surgical ward, one to the gynaecology ward and one to an orthopaedic ward. Despite these outliers, an ICP was completed for all patients (33/33) from the time of admission to their day of discharge.

Standards of care. Standards of between 97% and 100% were achieved for all patients for 6 of the 8 audit indicators as defined by the BTS 'audit of acute severe asthma' minimum data set. A standard of 91% was achieved for one of the remaining indicators and 70% for the other (*see* Table 9.4).

(1) Assessment on admission

The trust recorded peak expiratory flow (PEF) significantly more often than other hospitals reporting in the 1995 National Audit. The trust also performed blood gases on admission no less often and systemic steroids were prescribed significantly more often than these other hospitals.

Table 9.4 Standards of care indicators

Indicator	1991–92 national audit (34 centres) (N = 900) (%)	1995 national audit (34 centres) (N = 1508) [%(n)]	Trust (N = 33) [%(n)]	Chi-square	P value	Fisher's exact P value
PEF measured	83	88 (1325)	100 (33)	4.544	**0.033**	**0.026**
PCO$_2$ recorded	69	69 (1043)	70 (23)	0.004	0.948	1.000
Systemic steroids given	86	75 (1129)	91 (30)	6.001	**0.014**	**0.012**
PEF variability recorded	78	77 (1159)	97 (32)	7.442	**0.006**	**0.003**
Inhaled steroids given on discharge	80	85 (1288)	97 (32)	3.512	0.061	0.075
Oral steroids given on discharge	78	81 (1215)	97 (32)	5.625	**0.018**	**0.013**
OPD appointment given	73	65 (987)	100 (33)	17.225	**<0.001**	**<0.001**
Self-management plan given	11	27 (414)	97 (32)	75.882	**<0.001**	**<0.001**

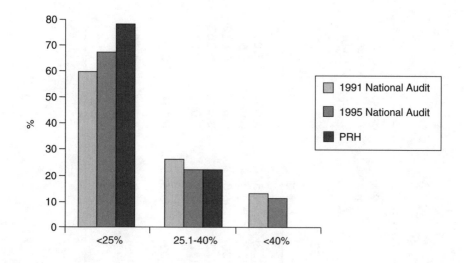

Figure 9.1 Level of peak expiratory flow variability at discharge.

(2) Management in hospital in all ward areas

The trust recorded PEF variability in the 24 hours prior to discharge in 97% (32/33) of cases, significantly more often than other hospitals reporting in the 1995 audit. No patients were discharged from the hospital with a peak expiratory flow variability of more than 40%; this is illustrated in Figure 9.1.

(3) Discharge from hospital

The trust sent the majority of patients home with inhaled steroids (in line with the centres in the 1995 national audit) but more patients were discharged with oral steroids. The trust was signifi-cantly better at sending patients home with a follow-up out-patient appointment and a self-management plan. For 30 (90%) of patients the appointment was with a consultant in respiratory medicine. This is illustrated in Figure 9.2.

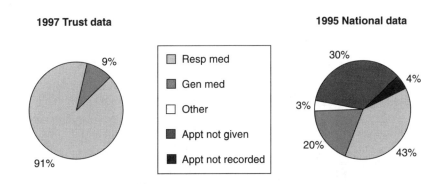

Figure 9.2 Type of discharge planned.

Education for staff. The amount of educational support provided is shown in Table 9.5.

Table 9.5 Educational support provided

Professional group	Nurses, PAMS	Doctors	CNS respiratory care
Time	30 hours	3 hours	14.5 days
Number	82	10	1
Locations	PGMC, wards, OPD	Medical department	998 in house, St Mary's and conference centre
Costs	None	None	£245

User satisfaction with information received. During February, 14 patients attended a CNS follow-up appointment. All of these agreed to complete the questionnaires (*see* Figure 9.3).

Overall, users responded favourably regarding satisfaction with information received. 78% (11/14) reported that they had either received about the right amount or too much information about four of the key areas identified, namely:

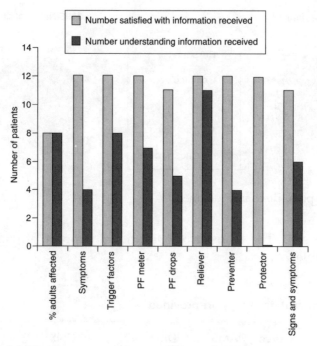

Figure 9.3 Responses to patient questionnaires.

- What are the main symptoms of asthma?
- What is meant by an asthma trigger factor?
- How to use a peak flow meter
- Which medicine is a protector, a reliever or a preventer?

In relation to the same four key areas many of the users were unable to demonstrate an understanding of the information received. Fewer than 30% (4/14) were able to describe their symptoms of asthma and none of them could name their protector. However, the numbers are too small to derive any statistical significance.

Conclusions

Improvements in quality of patient care

Improvements in all key standards of patient care were identified. These included improvements in the areas highlighted at the beginning of the project, particularly safe discharge and appro-priate specialist follow-up. Knowledge and skills of staff have been extended through workshops, ward-based groups and one-to-one sessions, and sessions for doctors. Evidence of the success of this educational approach is the completion of the asthma ICP for all patients, regardless of the type of admitting ward, and the subse-quent high standards of care achieved.

User education and self-management

One of the aims of the project was to improve patients' under-standing about their asthma and provide written information for self-management. However, the results suggest that whilst most patients (97%) were given a written self-management plan and associated education this was not indicative of individual satisfaction or understanding. These results raise questions, including (a) what is the best approach to providing information/education?, and (b) when is the most appropriate time to deliver it? The project team concluded that an adequate strategy for education could not be achieved in isolation from primary care services and must consider the input of both practice nurses and GPs. However, we must first understand what individual beliefs and perceptions may influence satisfaction and understanding before any strategy can be developed.

Project limitations

It has not been possible to identify longer term outcomes from this one-year project. Many of these outcomes require a research approach. The impact on readmissions and acute attendances, for example, could only be assessed over a number of years.

The method for surveying user satisfaction was limited. Issues of self-presentational bias had not been addressed and the third questionnaire 'What do you understand about your asthma?' has not been validated. However, the suggestion that a disparity exists between satisfaction with information received and what has been understood is strong enough to support investigating these issues through a formal research programme.

Reflection

A number of key learning points have been highlighted throughout the process of implementing guidelines within a formal framework. These include:

1 Project management

   - have a clear project plan and timeframe from the outset

   - each member of the team should know their responsibilities in relation to the project

   - keep on target, do not get sidetracked

   - clearly identify outcome measures at the outset.

2 Multi-professional working

   - ensure the early establishment of MPT steering group and meet on a regular basis

   - value each others' roles.

3 Change management

   - ensure ownership by relevant professional groups

   - be flexible, adapt to culture and unpredicted pressures

   - user involvement helps.

Plans for the future

The completion of this project must be viewed as achieving improvements for one part of the patient care pathway only. The aim for good asthma management should be to achieve a complete care pathway between primary care and the hospital and back to primary care again.

A second project, 'The community link project', has been proposed by the trust and funding awarded by the health authority. The work will be undertaken by the existing Respiratory CNS through secondment to the Clinical Effectiveness Department and supported by a steering group.

Audit of acute severe asthma in hospital will continue and be extended to include primary care management of asthma.

Part 3

10

Reaching general conclusions from specific projects

CAROL DUMELOW AND PETER LITTLEJOHNS

In this chapter we explore whether any general lessons can be learnt from looking at each project in detail. At the end of the year Peter Littlejohns interviewed each project leader. The interviews were recorded and qualitative analysis by another researcher (Carol Dumelow) was undertaken. We describe in detail the methods, results and conclusions.

Methods of analysis

The six interviews were tape recorded and transcribed verbatim. 'Framework' qualitative data analysis methods were used to analyse the interview data. 'Framework' is a technique developed by the Social and Community Planning Research Unit for applied qualitative research (Ritchie and Spencer, 1994). It is an analytical process which has been developed specifically for applied policy research using qualitative data collection methods. Qualitative methods in applied policy research broadly answer four types of questions: (i) contextual; (ii) diagnostic; (iii) evaluative; or (iv) strategic (Ritchie and Spencer, 1994). Research which attempts to address evaluative questions will ask the following types of questions.

Evaluative: appraising the effectiveness of what exists

For example (Ritchie and Spencer, 1994, p.174),

- How are objectives achieved?
- What affects the successful delivery of programmes or services?
- How do experiences affect subsequent behaviours?
- What barriers exist to systems operating?

Since the interview data from the ACE project was both evaluative in nature and had a pre-defined framework of questions to be answered, it was considered appropriate to use 'Framework' qualitative analysis techniques. The first part of this chapter will provide a detailed description of 'Framework' qualitative data analysis methods. The latter part will discuss the findings from the ACE project. The analytic approach used involved six stages (*see* Figure 10.1).

The first stage of the analysis involved reading the transcripts to gain an overview of the information gathered during the interviews and to identify recurrent themes and key issues prevalent in the interview data. Following on from this initial stage, a thematic framework was developed (*see* Table 10.1) which contained nine categories: (i) measuring patient outcomes; (ii) use of guidelines; (iii) user involvement; (iv) education and training for professionals and users; (v) education and training for project co-ordinators; (vi) collaboration; (vii) project management; (viii) timing; and (ix) impact of project on changing practice. These categories reflect the topic areas and questions covered during the interviews, together

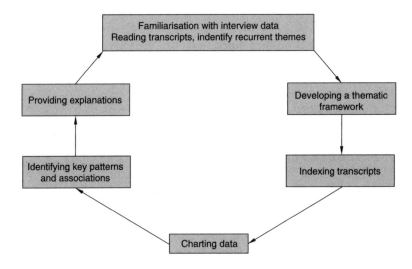

Figure 10.1 An overview of 'framework' qualitative data analysis methods.

with additional categories which emerged from the interview data.

The third stage of the analysis involved indexing the interview transcripts. The numerical coding system outlined in the thematic framework was systematically applied to the interview text. Codes were assigned to each part of the interview text and were written in the margins of the six interview transcripts (*see* Table 10.2).

The fourth stage of the analysis involved charting the data. The aim of this stage of the analysis was to build a picture of the whole data, including the range of responses for each issue. A number of charts, containing headings and sub-headings, were developed, which were drawn from the thematic framework. For each respondent, the appropriate sections of the indexed interview transcript were summarised and written on to the relevant chart (*see* Table 10.3). Numerically ordered identification codes were used to identify respondents and were ordered in the same way for each chart. This enabled analysis between and across respondents.

The final stage of analysis involved reviewing the charts to identify key patterns and associations within the interview data. These patterns and associations were used during the final stage of

Table 10.1   The thematic framework developed from the interview data (extract)

1   Measurement of patient outcomes
       1.1 Patient outcomes chosen
       1.2 Process of identifying patient outcomes
       1.3 Reasons for selecting patient outcomes
       1.4 Patient outcomes achieved
       1.5 Patient outcomes to be measured post project timetable
       1.6 Own attitude towards measuring patient outcomes
       1.7 Problems experienced measuring patient outcomes

2   Use of clinical guideline
       2.1 Reasons for choice of guideline
       2.2 Process used to apply guideline to local setting
       2.3 Problems with applying guideline to local practice
       2.4 Factors enabling guideline to be applied locally
       2.5 Attitude towards using clinical guideline
       2.6 Problems experienced choosing a guideline
       2.7 Changes made to guideline
       2.8 Result of the localisation process

3   User involvement
       3.1 Type of user involvement
       3.2 Problems with user involvement
       3.3 Benefits of user involvement
       3.4 Attitude of users towards programme
       3.5 Attitude towards involving users

the analysis to provide a model by which guidelines could be successfully implemented within a clinical setting. The next section will discuss the key findings from the ACE project interviews.

Results

The six pilot projects had variable success in implementing their guidelines within the remit of the ACE project. The majority of

Table 10.2 Example of an indexed transcript

Resp:	One of the keys things probably is you've got to do your homework right at the beginning. You've really got to find out what's going on out there so you tailor your programme to meet any needs, otherwise you meet barriers. Right at the very beginning, or if you do meet barriers, you recognise them and find your way around them.	10.7 factors contributing to success
	Well we knew right from the beginning that the GPs were a potential barrier so we sidestepped them to a certain extent and got round them that way. From the nurses' perspective, education and training seems to be very critical. We very strongly believe in the training and education side. We found, they probably found it more important having a facilitator who is there. We actually went round with a facilitator of the project. It wouldn't have worked without.	10.5 difficulties overcome 4.2 support needed 7.2 importance of a key worker
Int:	Would you like to add anything to that?	
Resp:	No I don't think so. I think the biggest thing that I found and at times it was disappointing, was this inability to change people at certain levels of their career.	9.9. attitude towards changing practice

pilot projects had adapted national or local guidelines for use in their clinical setting and had identified one or two patient outcomes which they intended to measure. Five out of the six projects considered they had been successful in achieving guideline implementation within their chosen clinical setting; however, levels

Table 10.3 Example of a chart developed during the analysis

Chart 3: user involvement

Respondent	3.1 Type of user involvement	3.2 Problems with user involvement	3.3 Benefits of user involvement	3.4 Attitude of users towards programme	3.5 Attitude of project managers towards involving users
001	Involved in meetings, evaluation, presenting results				
002	In-depth interviews				
003	Representative on Steering Group				
004	In-depth interviews with users				
005	Interviews with patients				
006	Representative on Steering Group				

of success varied within these five projects. One project had not been successful and at the time of interview was in the early stages of guideline implementation. Analysis of the interview data highlighted clear patterns across the six pilot projects regarding the factors needed to implement guidelines successfully within a clinical setting. Six themes were identified as important factors contributing towards successful guideline implementation which have been categorised into the following areas: (i) education, training and support; (ii) user involvement; (iii) multi-professional collaboration; (iv) professional environment; (v) effective project management; and (vi) organisation of guideline implementation. The remainder of this chapter will discuss these themes in greater detail.

Education, training and support

Education and training for professionals and users was a key aspect of the guideline implementation process for five out of the six projects. Two types of education and training took place: (i) seminars and study days for professional groups; and (ii) training within clinical settings. Education was considered to be an important aspect of the guideline implementation process, particularly for nurses or ward staff responsible for managing change in working practice.

> *setting up two hour sessions with the district nurses at their base and out in the practices and then throughout the implementation processes this continued together with training on the spot ... from the nurses' perspective, education and training seems to be very critical.* (**002, Pilot Site, Project Manager**)

A second aspect was the education and training needed for the project managers leading the ACE pilot projects. Access to advice and training from experts in the field on guidelines and outcome measurement was an important factor. However, additional training on how to measure patient outcomes effectively was needed. This highlights the need for professional staff within clinical settings to have access to academic units, which can provide specialist knowledge and advice on the process of implementing guidelines.

User involvement

One theme evident amongst the ACE pilot projects was the issue of user involvement. A key problem experienced was obtaining appropriate user involvement in the guideline implementation process. Obtaining user involvement by means of participation on steering groups or by focus group was not successful. Problems arose with identifying appropriate patients to represent users' views, getting active participation at meetings and difficulties getting patients to attend meetings. The most successful approach had been through involvement on a one-to-one basis with users, typically by interview with a sample of patients.

> *I don't think our user focus group worked terribly well. In my inital bit, trying to set it out with a few patients, I found that there was so much arguing between patients and keeping them to the point was a little bit difficult and I think they preferred getting an in-depth interview on their own. I would do it the same way again.* **(002 Pilot Site, Project Manager)**

> *We have got a couple of users on placements on the steering group; of which one has been a fairly regular attender. They have been terribly passive at the moment. I am not sure it is the right setting to involve him and I suspect it is probably better that involvement of users should perhaps be in terms of the actual intervention they are getting and getting feedback from how helpful they find things.* **(006 Pilot Site, Project Manager)**

The benefit of user involvement in the guideline implementation process was evident amongst all six pilot projects. Importantly, gaining information from a user's perspective of the service had provided new insights and a different perspective from the professionals running the service.

> *It made me realise that my perceptions were not the same as*

patient's perceptions ... Patients didn't seem to remember anything they had been told about health education, about discussing their leg ulcer or the outcomes or anything ... they couldn't remember it so we were doing something wrong. So this led us to query how to put messages across. **(004, Pilot Site, Project Manager)**

It was also very useful for ward staff, nursing staff and doctors to hear the opinions of the users and to understand what it is actually like to use the service here. And they provide a very useful insight actually ... very constructive comments. **(001, Pilot Site, Project Manager)**

Multi-professional collaboration

Collaboration between different professional groups was a key factor during the guideline implementation process. Levels of collaboration varied across the pilot projects but all project managers considered they had received the level of collaboration they required. Managers in provider trusts and health commissioners had a passive involvement in most projects whereby they provided support for the project but were not directly involved. The pilot projects that sought collaboration with GPs had variable support from GPs for the project. One pilot project collaborated with an academic unit to provide expertise in measuring patient outcomes. Overall, all six pilot projects considered multi-professional working had led to improved working relationships between different professional groups and had been beneficial in aiding the process of guideline implementation.

Multi-professional working can really happen and can be very successful and I think one of the keys to that is to be aware or be open to the issue that there is a balance of skills and perspectives and that you have to value each other's role. So it's not trying to ensure that everybody is doing the same thing; people might be doing different things but seeing how they balance and how they work together and having respect for those with different contributions. **(001, Pilot Site, Project Manager)**

I think what has been a bit more useful across the differing disciplines, is bringing them together and having to agree a strategy on how some of these interventions could be offered ... whilst before I think it was being sort of excessively eclectic in their approach, almost in a sense not knowing quite what they are going to do when you send someone over there. So I think it's been helpful in that sense. **(006, Pilot Site, Project Manager)**

Professional environment

The professional environment within which the guideline was implemented was important in leading to the success of the project. Four out of the six pilot ACE projects identified the timing of the funding as instrumental to the success of the project. This was primarily because the clinical area in which the guideline was to be implemented had been highlighted as a priority area prior to funding being provided, which was associated in many cases with both involvement of professionals at an early stage of the project design and their enthusiasm towards ensuring the guideline was implemented. Ownership of the project was a key theme in contributing towards its success, whereby all professionals involved had a shared objective and a commitment towards the project. In two of the pilot projects a project plan had already been identified which had contributed to the success of these projects within the set time-scale.

The project actually came from enthusiasts within the hospital. It was decided that they wanted to tackle it and it was just timely that there was the ACE funding there to do it. **(001 Pilot Site, Project Manager)**

It was quite happy timing because the gynaecology department had already decided that they wanted to look at this so it's sort of correct timing. **(005, Pilot Site, Project Manager)**

All the members of the steering group have kept very close to the project and have stayed very enthusiastic about it throughout but I think that's because they've been all involved in writing the integrated care pathway. **(001, Pilot Site, Project Manager)**

Effective project management

Success in achieving guideline implementation within the remit of the ACE project was influenced by the project management approach adopted. While clear milestones and time-scales were essential in monitoring the progress of the project, flexibility towards unpredicted pressures within the clinical setting was also important. In particular, flexibility in being able to foresee or overcome barriers within the clinical setting.

We were flexible enough to adapt to the culture that we are in here. Faced with unpredicted pressures we still kept on target and didn't get side-tracked at all. **(001, Pilot Site, Project Manager)**

One of the key things probably is that you've got to do your homework right at the beginning. You've really got to find out what's going on out there so that you tailor your programme to meet any needs, otherwise you meet barriers. Or if you do meet barriers you recognise them and find your way around them. **(002, Pilot Site, Project Manager)**

Managing guideline implementation was successful when clear milestones were set within a defined time-scale. However, the length of time needed to implement a guideline and assess the outcome of this intervention on patients was highly dependent upon the area of clinical practice chosen and was not always feasible within the set time-scale of the ACE project. Problems were experienced by some pilot projects in measuring the patient outcomes they had identified within a time-scale of one year.

Organisation of guideline implementation

Two key themes were evident amongst the pilot projects concerning the organisation of guideline implementation. First, the role of a key worker to provide project management and support and encouragement to staff involved in the guideline implementation. Secondly, the need for continuity within the guideline implementation process. This second theme was closely linked with changing professional practice issues.

The role of a key worker to provide on-going education and support to staff involved in the guideline implementation was a key factor within two of the pilot projects. In both projects, this role was considered instrumental in ensuring the guideline was implemented.

What we've found is getting a multi-professional team together but have a clinical nurse specialist actually driving them. I would suspect that if you took the clinical nurse specialist out, the project wouldn't survive as well ... to really drive it, to provide the on-going education, to supply knowledge and the support one-to-one to ward staff. **(001, Pilot Site, Project Manager)**

We found they probably found it more important having a facilitator who is there. We actually went round with a facilitator of the project. It wouldn't have worked without ... you've got to keep tying up loose ends and encouraging them. **(002, Pilot Site, Project Manager)**

Continuity within the guideline implementation process was a key theme amongst the six pilot projects. Five pilot projects had been successful in creating change in working practices as a result of implementing a guideline within a specific clinical setting. However, maintaining this change in working practice once the project was complete and funding had ended is a key issue. Four project managers considered that their project had been successful in producing a lasting change in working practice, but there was some concern that further improvement in working practice was unlikely without continued support for the professional staff involved. However, various initiatives were planned by these project managers to ensure current working practices were maintained.

The process developed during the ACE project to implement guidelines within a clinical setting was considered by three pilot projects to have provided a model to apply to other clinical areas.

One project manager was doubtful that the work gained through the project would be sustained if a more permanent infrastructure for guideline implementation was not developed. This highlights the problem that exists with the current arrangements in healthcare services for implementing guidelines. Although models such as the ACE projects enable guidelines to be implemented within individual clinical settings, there is a need for this process to be applied to other clinical areas with an infrastructure to support this on a much wider scale.

We need an infrastructure here to do this sort of thing. This is about making one guideline. To do this properly we should have been working this guideline up for say a year. We might have spent a year focusing rather hard on it, which in this case we have done, but then there is follow-up work and it will need looking at in six months time to see if it is still going on, but in parallel to that we should be doing something on the GI cancer or bleed. Unless we take the sort of approach we have taken here and say this works so well that the organisation will provide the same resources towards making us a standing issue for the department if they want someone permanently, then it is sort of dropped into the wilderness and lost. **(003, Pilot Site, Project Manager)**

I think it probably is an effective way of doing it. I think we probably need a lot of projects for it to have much impact and perhaps what we need to try to do is to get key people to work in a slightly more regional way, beyond their own trust. **(006, Pilot Site, Project Manager)**

Experience from the ACE projects suggests that at present, guideline implementation seems to be an *ad-hoc* process instituted by the enthusiastic individual practitioner, rather than a strategic approach supported by management and co-ordinated within the contracting process. In summary, the themes discussed in this chapter that were evident amongst the six ACE pilot projects provide a model by which guidelines can be successfully implemented in individual clinical settings (*see* Figure 10.2). This model could provide a framework to enable guidelines to be implemented in a more generic sense.

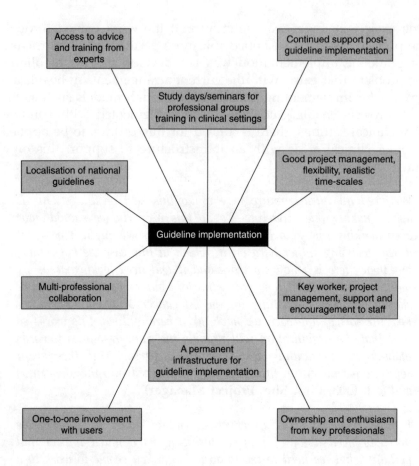

Figure 10.2 Factors contributing to successful guideline implementation.

11

The second and third years of ACE

ACE II

On the basis of the perceived success of the first year, a second year of funding was made available. The process of resource allocation was the same as in year 1, with the addition of a Buddy scheme between ACE I and ACE II sites. Panel members were:

Lyn Harris, Senior Project Officer, R&D South Thames RO

Professor Peter Littlejohns, Director, HCEU

Dr Marcia Kelson, College of Health

Stephen Fash, Chief Executive, St Peter's Hospital NHS Trust

Dr Patrick Bower, GP, Balham

Dr Lois Lodge, Consultant, Public Health, South Thames RO

Debra Humphris, Programme Leader

Table 11.1 ACE II 1997–98, successful sites

Site	Guideline topic
Eastbourne and County Health Care NHS Trust	Implementation of guidelines to promote the uptake and maintenance of breast feeding
Kingston and District Community NHS Trust	Implementing a pressure area care clinical guideline
Mid Kent Health Care NHS Trust	Treatment and follow-up of patients with hepatitis C
North Downs Community NHS Trust	Implementation of guidelines for the management of childhood asthma
Pathfinder Mental Health Services NHS Trust	Implementation of guidelines for the assessment of side-effects of antipsychotics in the maintenance and treatment of schizophrenia
The Royal West Sussex NHS Trust	Implementation of local guidelines for the management of secondary hyperlipidaemia
East Sussex, Brighton and Hove Health Authority	Implementation of clinical guidelines on the management of low back pain in general practice

At the same time, the region commissioned an external evaluation of the first two years of the ACE Programme. The results are available as a separate report (*see* p. 145). The successful sites were as shown in Table 11.1.

ACE III

Building on the experience of the first two years, a third year of the ACE Programme was developed. The emphasis changed slightly as it aimed to create an evaluative culture within the NHS organisation from the boardroom to the bedside. In order that trust and health authority boards could provide this leadership, the additional element of ACE III is an Executive Learning Set in which two key individuals responsible for clinical effectiveness at board level within the organisation, one executive and one non-executive, will participate and support the project within their organisation. Through this approach it is anticipated that the programme will enable both operationally and strategically the development of a culture that systematically manages knowledge into practice. The aims for ACE III have been identified as:

(a) The development of capacity at executive board level to provide direction to the development of an evaluative culture within NHS organisations.

(b) Strategic leadership by two board members within the NHS organisation on the issue of clinical effectiveness.

(c) The implementation, by clinicians, of the findings of specific robust research evidence with active managerial involvement and support.

Again, bids were invited against specific criteria. The panel consisted of:

Professor Peter Littlejohns, Director, HCEU

Dr Marcia Kelson, College of Health

Dr Lois Lodge, Consultant, Public Health South Thames RO

Dr Terry Desombre, University of Surrey

Debra Humphris, Programme Leader

ACE III criteria

• The area of clinical concern selected should have potential for improving specific patient outcomes locally and be agreed by both purchaser and provider before commencement.

- The evidence to be implemented must be robust and have been critically appraised.

- All proposals must include a clear project plan with objectives, time-scales, financial details and management arrangements. Where possible these arrangements should link with the health authority, and appropriate regional office involvement.

- Proposals must demonstrate collaborative inter-professional working. Consideration must also be given to working across the range of appropriate interfaces and sectors.

- Implementation should take an educational approach.

- Outcome measures must be identified based on the evidence source to be implemented and linked to the trust's clinical audit programme.

The successful sites are shown in Table 11.2.

Table 11.2 Successful sites in ACE III

Site	Guideline topic
Ashford & St Peter's Hospitals NHS Trust	The management of chronic obstructive pulmonary disease
Lambeth, Southwark & Lewisham Multi-professional Audit Research Group	Treatment of depression in primary care
Merton, Sutton & Wandsworth Health Authority	Ensuring appropriate referral and investigation of patients with suspected colorectal cancer
Oxleas NHS Trust	The management of imminent violence
University Hospital Lewisham	Intercollegiate Stroke Audit

On-going evaluation

Each of the ACE sites is required to provide a final and full report against their project objectives. As well as detailing of the pre- and post-audit data, and the nature of their educational interventions, project teams are encouraged to maintain a reflective journal about the process they have undertaken. Often the most powerful learning from such a process cannot be captured in audit data alone, so teams are encouraged to include their reflections on the experience of implementing the guideline.

External evaluation

For ACE III, with the added dimension of the board members' involvement, an external evaluator has been commissioned to explore with this group a range of issues related to managing knowledge into practice, both before and after the process. Each individual will be interviewed, using a semi-structured question-naire. Interviews will be taped and transcribed.

Interviews will explore specifically where the board member assesses the organisation to be at the start of the project, in relation to use of research evidence, and how they anticipate their own role and the role of the trust board in facilitating the management of research knowledge into practice. Thirdly, they will be asked what they consider to be the critical conditions necessary at a strategic level to support the promotion of evidence-based, clinical practice. This process will be repeated at the end of the project.

12

The ACE start-up framework

DEBRA HUMPHRIS

Implementing a clinical guideline, as with any change in management process, requires preparation. To assist you with that process the following framework presents a number of stages you should consider before starting. It is by no means exhaustive, and you may want to add points as you progress.

Where are you now?

- Take time to assess and reflect upon the situation into which you seek to introduce change.

- Be clear about why you want to do this and you what the desired outcomes are.

- What are the links to and with the wider organisation, both operational and strategic.

Guideline development

- Are you clear about the quality of the guideline that you want to implement?

- Have you considered the consequences of the quality of the guideline?

Implementation strategy

- Involve all the key stakeholders at an early stage.
- Develop a clear and realistic, week-by-week implementation plan.
- Build in points at which you systematically monitor your progress.
- Communication is critical, try to knit into existing channels, use a range of methods.
- Do not underestimate the hidden costs.
- Plan carefully the educational approach and provision to fit to appropriate audiences.
- You may want to set a launch data to mark the formal start.
- Dissemination via postal distribution is often ineffective, wherever possible use an interactive approach.
- The credibility of the facilitator of the change can have a considerable bearing upon the outcome.

Patient/user involvement

- Consider how to involve appropriate user groups, this may be more appropriate than a single patient.
- You should consider the need for training and costs in terms of time and travel.

Organisational systems

- Knowing the organisation is important, try to fit the changes into existing systems.

- Make clear links with the organisation's wider quality framework and arrangements for clinical governance.

- Involve, or keep informed, the board members with responsibility for quality and effectiveness.

- The more boundaries, professional and oganisational, that you cross the more complex managing the process becomes.

Sustainability

- Begin to think as you plan the implementation about sustaining the improvements you achieve.

- Remember that all guidelines have a shelf life, do you know the review date?

- How will you lock in the learning from the process and use it to good effect again?

Learning needs

- The implementation of the guideline may identify learning needs that will need to be addressed.

- Critical appraisal skills should be developed in all those involved in the process.

- Change in management skills should be developed in all those involved in the process.

13

External evaluation of the ACE initiative

CAROLYN MILLER, JULIE SCHOLES AND PEGGY FREEMAN

At the end of the first year of the ACE Programme, the South Thames NHS Executive commissioned an independent study to evaluate the initiative. The evaluation was to include 13 sites: the six first-round sites and seven second-round sites. This chapter discusses some of the challenges presented by the evaluation, the methods used by the evaluation team and finally, a summary of the key findings.[1]

The evaluators were commissioned to discover what factors distinguished a successful ACE site; and second, to determine the effects of a 'buddy' system, which was introduced for the second round of the ACE projects. The idea of the buddies was that those people involved in the first round of projects would contribute their experience to the project personnel in the second round by acting as advisers to them.

---

[1] A detailed account of the findings can be found in the Appendix to this chapter.

The immediate question for the evaluation team to explore was: what was meant by a *successful* ACE site and on what criteria? It was obvious from the start that each ACE project was different in scope, in its aims, in the number of people involved and in the origin of the guideline. Further exploration showed that projects also had different starting points, some beginning almost from scratch and others working from an already prepared base. Some projects appeared to have more 'difficult' situations or more challenging people to win over if they were to get the guidelines implemented: getting a key 'gate keeper' on board might be a significant success for one project but not as crucial for another.

This variation between the projects led to the conclusion that a meaningful appraisal of the criteria on which 'success' could be gauged had to come from illuminating the situations in which the projects were trying to succeed. The sponsors of the evaluation appreciated this contextual variation, while at the same time looking for clarity and measurable success factors which could be generalisable to other situations. There is often a tension between the desire for generalisable indicators, which can be applied to a large number of settings, and the knowledge that it is the variables within each context which can be the key to whether an innovation works or not. For a long time this has been at the centre of much debate about evaluation methodologies: what may be generalisable may not be specific enough to be useful when applied to another setting.[2] The approach we adopted to evaluating 13, very different, projects was:

1 to research each of the ACE projects as a *case study*
2 then to take the issues about guideline implementation which

---

[2] For example, in evaluation innovation in education during the 1970s, MacDonald *et al.* (1971) developed case study methodology to respond to his findings that the same innovation had quite different responses and outcomes in different schools. At about the same time, Parlett and Hamilton (1972), and Stake (1972) in the US, were developing similar models. All of these models have been drawn on in our methodology. Papers by these authors and full references can be found in *Beyond the Numbers Game: a reader in educational evaluation*. D Hamilton, D Jenkins, C King *et al.* (1977) Macmillan Education, London.

had arisen from the cases studies and *compare them across all cases*, looking at similarities, differences and unique circumstances

3 and finally to analyse the various issues in the implementation strategies and their outcomes in terms of a *profile of attributes* which act together to contribute to positive outcomes for guideline implementation. We included the potential for sustainability of the guideline's use after the end of the project as one of these attributes of its 'success'.

The first step for each case study was to find out how the different people taking part in the project experienced it, the activities they undertook and the organisational structure(s) they worked in so as to:

• assess the *starting point of the project* to give baseline data

• chart the *process of implementation* and the developments arising from the project

• identify the *organisational barriers and levers* which affected the implementation process

• from the baseline data, to identify the *'value added'* elements associated with participation in the project, including any changes and improvements in patient care

• collate *stakeholders' criteria for success* of the project

• assess the *role of the buddy* (for ACE II sites).

Data were collected by interviewing the project personnel who were the key players in the project, as well as other stakeholders who were influenced by the project. We attended events such as education sessions to launch a guideline and examined documentary data produced, including any audit material.[3] We did not

---

[3] We found that, in general, the audit data had a limited value in evaluating the outcomes of projects. This was because they tended to measure what was most easily measurable or because the statistics used did not quite reflect the scope or aims of the project.

collect audit data ourselves – that was the job of the projects' co-ordinators and would have been beyond the scope of a one-year evaluation.

In the next stage of drawing together data from all projects, we analysed topics such as:

- the way projects had been chosen in the first place
- reasons for introducing the guideline and its status
- the scale and complexity of the project
- what the funding had purchased (and some of the hidden costs)
- the different strategies people had employed for dissemination, education and implementation of the guidelines
- client/patient involvement
- organisational issues which had helped and hindered the process
- the operation of the buddies
- the different perspectives on what constituted success.[4]

In reviewing all this material in order to describe and explain the nature of the programme as a whole, the variety of circumstances faced by project personnel was clearly in evidence. It was very challenging for the evaluation team to make sense of 13 different projects, especially as ACE II sites were being visited on several occasions in order to cover various stages of the implementation process. At the same time, we were comparing data with the ACE I sites, who had already completed their projects. An additional complicating factor was that some of the ACE II projects had delayed the start of their initiative, for a variety of reasons. This meant that these project personnel had not gathered all the relevant audit data or finalised their report by the end of the year in which our evaluation had to finish. The result was that the evaluation team were still having to gather data right up to the end of the year, at the same time as drafting the evaluation report.

---

[4] It was interesting to find that all projects saw themselves as being 'successful' but used different criteria to come to that judgement. For some, completing the project was their main criterion.

The steering group appointed to the evaluation were clearly at times baffled and frustrated by this research process, which was not clear-cut, where hypotheses were being formed throughout and data were not made explicit because triangulation was incomplete.[5] But gradually a picture began to emerge of how project personnel handled different stages of the implementation process and coped with the range of problems along the way. It was not until the final part of the evaluation was reached, at the end of the year, that we were able to crystallise the key factors and to show how each contributed to the outcomes. Although the evaluation methodology was demanding and time consuming, it had shown, through a process of successive analyses, what the significant elements were in guideline implementation and the real world factors within each of the project contexts which enhanced or undermined the initiatives.[6]

In writing up the findings for the final report, we again found that the diversity of projects gave us cause for concern, this time in presenting the evidence. The usual research practice in reporting evidence from interviews is to select one or two 'typical' quotes from interviewees which illustrate the more general point; to use more quotations can soon make a report too long and can be repetitive. In this evaluation, one or two quotes were simply inadequate to portray the range of evidence for some of the issues being discussed. The imperative not to make the report unwieldy but to do justice to the range of responses from the different projects was unusually difficult in this case. The final report was pared down to 94 pages, plus an appendix. As for the two-page executive summary normally required by our sponsors, this was abandoned as it conveyed so little of the richness and diversity of the findings as to be almost meaningless to anyone wanting to know about implementing guidelines. Instead, we extracted the key points and summaries for each chapter of the report, its conclusions and

---

[5] This term derives from geological survey where different sight lines cross and is often used in research methodology to mean different data sources coming together to confirm or refute a piece of evidence or a hypothesis.

[6] The methodological procedures are rooted in Glaser and Strauss's method of constant comparative analysis, described in their influential book *The Discovery of Grounded Theory: strategies for qualitative research* (1967) Aldine, New York.

recommendations and compiled these into a synopsis. Although this does not convey people's experiences of projects in their own voices and nor does it give details about individual projects, it provides an accessible overview of the main issues. Readers are referred to the main report if they need to know more or want further information about the methods used to tackle the evaluation.

Appendix

Evaluation of the 'Assisting Clinical Effectiveness' Programme

Synopsis of final report

Carolyn Miller, Julie Scholes and Peggy Freeman

University of Brighton
Centre for Nursing and Midwifery Research

Report commissioned by;
NHSE South Thames
Project number: RDP 132

Start date: 1.5.97
End date: 30.4.98

Synopsis

This synopsis presents the key points in each chapter of the final report, ending with its conclusions and recommendations. The aim is to direct the reader to the various chapters of interest, to examine the evidence upon which these key points are made and to gain a more comprehensive account of the emergent issues. The summary points in the report are given as additional footnoted information in this synopsis.

1 Introduction

- This is an evaluation of 13 project sites implementing guidelines as part of an ACE initiative.

- The aim of the evaluation is to identify what made an 'ACE' site successful and in what way a buddy system facilitated the process.

- The evaluation methodology sought to capture the process as well as the outcomes of each initiative.

- The evaluation illuminates the common as well as idiosyncratic issues from the perspectives of the key stakeholders within each organisation.

2 Background to the use of guidelines

- There has been an explosion of information for the healthcare professions to assimilate. The evidence-based practice initiatives have attempted to distil the key issues from a wealth of literature and convey these in a straightforward and accessible way for clinicians to use.

- Evidence-based practice is seen to embody efficiency, effectiveness and quality. By determining specific ways to deliver care (based upon the 'best' scientific evidence) this can be construed as a criticism of healthcare professionals and a constraint on their autonomy.

- To get evidence into practice, clinicians and managers need to work collaboratively with systems which enable immediate access to relevant material/data for practice. One of the most effective ways of doing this is through the use of clinical guidelines.

- For guidelines to be effective, equal attention needs to be paid to the development, dissemination and implementation of the guideline.

- Patients/clients ought to be important partners in the guideline process, but who is involved and to what extent is variable according to the guideline and professional group implementing that guideline.

3 Methodology

- The stakeholder evaluation approach was used. Data were gathered by interview, documentary analysis and observation, and analysed by the constant comparative method.

- Data were gathered to cover three phases: baseline data, implementation processes and project outcomes.

- Interview reports and some of the draft conclusions were taken back to project facilitators for verification.

4 The projects and their guidelines

- The projects covered a diverse range of topics and had different agendas.

- Projects were chosen because: local 'opinion leaders' had a topic of particular interest; the publication of evidence stimulated local interest; a problem or shortfall in the standard of care had been identified; to make progress or diversify existing initiatives; or to capture local professional enthusiasm for a practice development.[1]

- There were considerable differences in the status of the guidelines and the evidence upon which they were based (e.g. three out of 13 guidelines used were based upon systematic reviews). Critical appraisal of the evidence upon which a guideline was based was weak.[2]

- A variety of tools were used to drive the guideline into practice. These included: integrated care pathways; assessments tools; a management plan' trust policy/protocols; and guidelines as flowcharts.

5 What did ACE funding buy?

- Projects varied in their funding from £7500 to £30 000.

---

[1] The nature of the evidence on which a guideline was based was variable to accommodate different topics and introduce guidelines to specialties that had previously not used them. A contradiction can be seen between the emphasis of what constitutes 'good evidence and good guidelines' espoused in the literature and the wish to see guidelines developed and used in clinical practice. When this was set beside definitions of clinical effectiveness, further contradictions emerged. Exceptions to the 'rule' had to be made to overcome the real world dilemmas of getting projects started and introducing guidelines to new disciplines.

[2] Some ACE projects were implemented on the basis of an individual judgement about the value and credibility of evidence in the literature. The methodological rigour and the extent to which the evidence was systematically and critically appraised was questionable (even though there was recognition of the importance of critical appraisal of the evidence). Many of the project facilitators indicated that the speed with which they had to prepare their proposals meant that, unless work in this area was in progress, critical evaluation occurred after submission of the proposal (and subsequently, in one case, not finding any evidence at all). This meant that some were not implementing national guidelines but generating their own. In other cases, people were accepting evidence or guidelines on the basis of the author's reputation or because the evidence appeared in a reputed professional journal. So the values espoused in the literature that the evidence underpinning the guidelines should be critically appraised and not based upon a single 'expert' opinion were contradicted in practice.

- The grant paid for: the dedicated time of the project facilitator; equipment necessary to run the project; and the opportunity to undertake an ACE programme with external learning support.[3]

- There was no direct relationship between the amount of the project grant and the complexity of each project.[4]

- Two elements contributed to the complexity of the project: the number of organisations involved and the number of disciplines targeted to use the guideline.

- The actual cost of the project was frequently underestimated, including the amount of time required to realise the project's ambitions and the seniority or level of experience required to make the project work.[5]

---

[3] In addition to funding personnel, the ACE package also provided learning support. The varied academic and professional backgrounds of the project facilitators meant that finding the right theoretical level and creating an appropriate learning environment to support the participants was complex. This generated mixed evaluations of the formal learning support days, and had an impact on enthusiasm and motivation in quite diametrically opposed ways. However, the consultation service offered by HECEU to project facilitators was highly valued.

One final thing that funding brought was kudos to the organisation from winning the project. This also contributed to the motivation and enthusiasm of the facilitators and raised their expectations to achieve the objectives of the project as well as to achieve the covert expectations of their colleagues on behalf of the organisation.

[4] It cannot be assumed that because a project sought to involve more than one organisation or discipline that it necessarily made the project more expensive (or better value for money) because the amount of work that had to be done was relative to the starting point of each organisation, the novelty of guidelines to the organisation and to the personnel expected to practise by them. Therefore, any immediate assumption of what is value for money should be tempered by caution and made after a careful examination of all the factors that make a project successful (see Section 10)

[5] ACE funding primarily paid for the dedicated time of a project facilitator. However, getting the right person in post within the constraints of the budget was a challenging activity or could generate hidden costs to the organisation if the grade of costs requirement was not estimated appropriately. Many of the project facilitators supplemented the bought time with work completed out of hours. Although ACE projects were funded by South Thames Regional Research and Development money, they were, in many cases, achieved and sustained by goodwill and enthusiasm.

- The clinical credibility and the match of professional background between the target professionals and the project facilitator was key to guideline implementation.[6]

- The target practitioners were significantly influenced by their perception of the project facilitator when making judgements about the merit of a guideline.[7]

6 The ACE process

- The ACE 'template' was baseline audit, introduction of a guideline with educational input and repeat audit.

- Phases in the guideline process were: development; dissemination; implementation; and evaluation.

- Although local adaptation of a national guideline encourages ownership and responsiveness to local patterns of working, there is a risk that too much change can counter the original research-based evidence.

- Face-to-face interaction coupled with continuing availability of the project facilitator were the most effective means of disseminating guidelines.[8]

---

[6] Given the importance of having the right person in post, the budget constraints sometimes meant delays to appointing a project facilitator or a revision of the original estimate of the whole-time equivalent that person could work on the project. The amount of responsibility and the overt and covert expectations on performance bore little relationship to clinical grading.

[7] Credibility seems to come more from the 'product sponsor' (project facilitator) rather than the independent credibility of the guideline. Many people adopted the guideline because of the project facilitator's endeavours, or because they wanted to assist the project facilitator. Face-to-face contact with practitioners was the most important interaction to get people enthusiastic about the guideline and the ACE project. Although the literature suggests that it is important for the project facilitator's disciplinary background to match the target practitioners, in a majority of cases the bid for the person undertaking the bulk of the work was based on a nursing salary scale. Doctors were paid for on a sessional basis.

[8] The most effective means of changing behaviour and sustaining practice, according to the guideline, was continued interaction with the project facilitator throughout the project. The implications of this on long-term sustainability are discussed in Chapter 6.

- The educational launch of the guideline should be tailored to the accustomed pattern of dissemination for each professional group.[9]

- One of the most effective prompts for guideline use was a locally adapted tool (e.g. Integrated Care Pathway/assessment tool), especially when this was supported by on-going interaction with the project facilitator.[10]

- Some elements of the audit included in the projects were simplistic and superficial, designed for ease of measurement rather than gaining a purchase on changed practice.

7 Patient/client involvement in guideline development

- All projects had a patient involved either as a member of the steering group or as evaluators of the service (post-guideline).[11]

[9] The education event or launch strategy was a key factor in determining the high, medium or low effect in reaching a number of practitioners and getting them to adopt the guideline. Launches by seminar or conference were successful in attracting a number of people, had the advantage of being less labour intensive (unless repeated on a number of occasions) but only reached people successfully who were interested enough to attend.

[10] There is insufficient evidence to identify which one of these strategies was definitely most effective. The approach taken to the guideline was dependent upon the context into which the guideline was to be placed and the practitioners it was to reach. However, the indicators are (from participant and stakeholder accounts) that the more effective development strategy was to use a national guideline adapted for use through an implementation tool. This is because practitioners pick up the tool every time they have contact with the patient group or use a national guideline unchanged but on a topic where there is pre-existing broad professional agreement about its content. The least successful developmental strategy was to circulate national or locally developed guidelines where there was local disagreement about the content.

[11] The majority of users were involved so as to gather their experience of their illness/treatment and convey this back to professionals, either through steering groups, working parties or by interview or questionnaires. In some cases, users were asked to ensure that written information that was disseminated was user friendly and understandable. In certain areas user involvement became more problematic because of the physical and mental health status of the patients. Some guidelines were considered to be too technical to involve patients in the process.

- When evaluating the patients' perspectives on the guidelines, people realised too late that ethical clearance should have been sought.

- The involvement of patients/clients ranged from token representation to active participation throughout the guideline process (when this was about patient guidelines).[12]

- Difficulties arose for patients and clinicians when involved with the steering group whilst undergoing treatment.

8 Organisational issues

- Barriers to implementation included: a negative perception of guidelines; assumptions about agreement of the guideline with underlying differences in interpretation and focus.[13]

- Resisters and blockers were more likely amongst those who worked independently and with a high level of professional autonomy. The reasons given were financial and time constraints.[14]

---

[12] Although the process of user involvement was recognised as problematic and the issues or representativeness of any one user acknowledged to be perplexing 'and probably beyond the remit of ACE' (PF HCEU: 22.11.97), users were expected to be involved to ensure that the 'guideline is sensitive to the views of those particular individuals' (PF HCEU: 22.11.97). On those criteria, either before, during or after the guideline was introduced, all the sites gauged the views of the users.

[13] Many of the barriers encountered when implementing the project were the reason why the project had been set up in the first place. Inconsistent practice, context-related difficulties, communicating within and across multi-disciplinary boundaries and across different organisations were the key challenges which had to be met.

[14] Gaining the participation of disparate groups of workers and trying to get them to work in a standard system generated resistance. In some cases this meant that project objectives had to be reformulated or alternative strategies adopted. Additional demands on fundholders' money caused some friction especially if this meant an additional outlay (even though in the long term this brought about financial benefits and improved client outcomes).

- The more organisations crossed by the guideline the weaker the penetration of the original message to the ultimate destination/ target professional group.

- Having a Trust Executive directly involved with the project was not seen to be an advantage in all but one case.[15]

- Levers to implementation: clinical credibility of the project facilitator who had a comprehensive knowledge of the organisation and the people who worked there; positional and legitimate authority or access to supportive personnel with that authority;[16] practical guidelines which facilitated practice.[17]

---

[15] All the project facilitators had either direct or indirect access to the executive board or senior managers within an organisation. Only one site felt the lack of trust authority behind the project had adversely influenced the outcome of their project. The initiatives were aimed at practitioners dealing with clinical matters and therein lay their strength and acceptability to practitioners. The site that had expressed difficulty, was the site that had problems getting GPs to fund the equipment and dressings needed to practice according to the guideline [as they disputed this should be paid for by the Community Trust rather than out of their funds]. But this issue raises an important point, that when or if guidelines are introduced that require an additional short-term expenditure, there needs to be agreement as to how that expenditure will be met before the guidelines are introduced.

[16] Significant levers included tapping into pre-existing systems within an organisation and using those systems to implement the ACE project. The project facilitator's clinical credibility or vicarious credibility by association with an opinion leader, was influential in encouraging recruitment to the project and the pooling or sharing of resources. However, when an ACE project was introduced into an environment without such systems in place, the project facilitator had to invest considerable time and effort in laying down those lines of communication and setting up collaborative working across different departments. In some sites all the project facilitator had to do was sow the seeds, whilst others were tilling fallow land. This significantly affected the time-scale by which all the ambitions of the project could be fulfilled.

[17] The quality and applicability of the guideline was a powerful lever. Having a robust guideline which could be seen to have direct benefit to the practitioner and their patient meant that much of the missionary work of selling or sponsoring the idea came from the project rather than the seller. The importance of professional relationships and knowing the organisation cannot be underestimated in its value to effect change and enable practitioners to respond positively to an ACE initiative.

9 Sustainability

- Sustainability can be defined in three ways: the project continues after funding;[18] the ACE approach becomes embedded into the organisation and is used to initiate other projects;[19] the learning that takes place through taking part in a project is applied to other work in the trust by the project facilitator.[20]

- A broader perspective on ACE would not only look at short-term but longer term outcomes, like sustainability.

- Although such evidence, by its nature, is speculative, there are indicators that predict that the long-term outcomes of a project are influenced by activities set in place whilst the project is in progress.

10 Defining success

- All project personnel saw their project as 'successful' according to their own criteria.

---

[18] Some projects were set up in the hope that funds would be made available to them once the ACE money had finished. Others saw this as a one-year initiative. In many instances the posts were funded at very low cost for a small component of the working week. However, when this project facilitator made a significant difference to the way practitioners worked in an organisation they were sorely missed (by patient and colleagues) when their role was discontinued along with external funding. Some sites were hoping to be able to gain internal funds by demonstrating the positive outcomes of the project. But their results came out at the end of the tight one-year programme (which had very little time to demonstrate change or sustainable change). They were therefore not in a bidding cycle that enabled them to put forward a convincing case to sustain or diversify the original project.

[19] The ACE template did seem to be taken up and translated to other topics and departments. But different organisations fostered different elements of the process which suited their clinical effectiveness strategy.

[20] One of the greatest losses to an organisation was the departure of a project facilitator appointed on a short-term contract. This also meant losing the collateral learning that the practitioner had gained by participating in the project. This suggests a lose lose situation for the Trust.

- The evaluators developed a framework made up of nine elements to examine the variables that had an impact upon projects. These were:

  1 Development of the guideline
  2 Dissemination strategy
  3 Education strategy
  4 Implementation strategy (prompts to get the practitioners to use the guideline)
  5 Patient/client involvement
  6 Organisational systems
  7 Sustainability of project
  8 Number of organisations crossed
  9 Impact upon practitioners

- The ultimate success of the project depended upon the interaction of each one of the elements.

- Each site adopted different strategies for each of the elements. Some of these strategies were more successful than others and were signified as such by the number of designated 'attributes' (maximum number 5). For example,

Elements	Attributes
Guideline development	◆◆
Education/launch	◆◆◆◆
Dissemination strategy	◆
Implementation strategy	◆
Patient/client involvement	◆◆◆
Organisational systems	◆◆◆◆
Sustainability	◆◆◆
No. organisations and disciplines	◆◆◆◆◆
Impact upon practitioners	◆

- The collective number of attributes were then banded.

Project	Total no. attributes	Banding
		A [41–45]
		B [36–40]
		C [31–35]
		D [26–30]
		E [21–25]
		F [16–20]
		G [11–15]
		H [6–10]

- The framework could be used as a tool to predict the likely outcome of a proposed project by assessing the number of attributes within the proposed approach to the guideline process and the pre-existing systems within the organisation.

- The collective number of attributes can then be banded to indicate the amount of time and money a project might require or the complexity of the project undertaken.

Project	Total no. attributes	Banding	
		A [41–45]	Increasing complexity
		B [36–40]	
		C [31–35]	
		D [26–30]	
		E [21–25]	
		F [16–20]	
		G [11–15]	
		H [6–10]	More time or money
		I [0– 5]	

11 Buddies

- Those who had experience of ACE projects in their first year were set up as buddies to support the practice facilitator on ACE sites in the second year (buddied).[21]

- The assumption that experience alone would be sufficient training for the role was not borne out in practice.[22]

- Matching academic and professional backgrounds and specific training to enhance facilitation skills was missing.[23]

- Lack of clarity about the role on both sides militated against a productive buddy relationship.[24]

- In some cases the buddies gained from the role because it enabled them to reflect back upon their project and consider

---

[21] The buddy system for the majority was unsuccessful.

[22] There had been an assumption that because a project facilitator had undertaken one ACE project they would be able to support someone in the second wave. However, the clinical and academic background of the buddies differed greatly as did their experience of project management and teaching. Therefore, the notion that one person's experience could inform another's because it had something to do with ACE was unrealistic.

[23] The time-scale of the project meant that the project facilitators wanted resolutions to problems fast. It took a great deal of effort to explain the project and the subcultural world in which it was set to outsiders who had no understanding of the organisational milieu. When time was short, such explanation was an additional burden contradicting the notion that the buddy was there to facilitate. When a buddy was matched by relative professional experience they were able to draw upon a common language and insight into the issues. In this situation the relationship worked to good effect. There was little that was common to any one project (apart from the theoretical notion of the ACE process). Each project facilitator encountered different barriers and levers within their organisation. The most important asset to the project facilitator was their insider knowledge of the organisation and the practitioners working there. If they did not know of someone personally they would use their own professional network to access an appropriate resource. The buddy, an outsider to the scenario, could not offer any such quick-fix solutions.

[24] The buddies might well have benefited from more formal training to help them with the role of facilitating others, giving constructive criticism and clarification over role boundaries. The circumstances in which the buddies first met could also have benefited from more time, a more informal atmosphere in which to discuss the issues.

future projects or topics in their trust by observing the work undertaken by the buddied.

12 Conclusions and recommendations

12.1 The evidence

The evidence on which a guideline was based was variable to accommodate different topics and introduce guidelines to specialities that had not previously used them. There is a hiatus between the rhetoric about guidelines and the reality of guideline development in practice.

Recommendation 12.1

When identifying an ACE site, there should be more emphasis placed upon establishing a minimum standard for the evidence to be developed into a guideline and scrutiny of the critical appraisal process of that evidence.

12.2 Critical appraisal of the evidence/ guideline

Some ACE projects were implemented on the basis of an individual judgement about the value and credibility of evidence in the literature. The methodological rigour and the extent to which the evidence was systematically and critically appraised was open to question. Clinicians appeared willing to accept a guideline because of the person who 'sponsored' its introduction. They assumed that critical appraisal of the evidence had gone before and that the guideline was credible without question (or with minor challenge).

Recommendation 12.2

Greater emphasis needs to be placed on developing critical

appraisal skills, specifically for the project facilitators, but also for the clinicians for whom the guideline is intended.

12.3 Value for money

One cannot assume that because a project sought to involve more than one organisation or discipline that it necessarily made the project more expensive (or better value for money). This was because the amount of work that had to be done was relative to the starting point of each organisation, the novelty of guidelines to the organisation and to the personnel expected to practise by them. However, the greater the number of organisational and disciplinary boundaries crossed the greater the complexity of the project and, unless adequately resourced, this could diminish the impact upon practitioners.

Recommendation 12.3

There needs to be a careful examination of the number of organisations and disciplines a project proposes to cross. These factors might well influence the amount of money requested to run a project, as more people would be required to match each discipline and organisation involved. However, there is no guarantee that this will produce better value for money or a greater number of positive outcomes from the project. This is more likely to be influenced by the time given to a project and the starting point of that organisation in terms of their previous work on guidelines. It would be helpful to identify a minimum benchmark based on a measure of the complexity of the project (as defined by the banding of attributes) by which a region considered a project to be value for money.

12.4 The project facilitator

The person appointed as project facilitator had more to do with matching the person's salary to fit the budget constraint rather than appointing the right person with sufficient positional and legitimate authority within the organisation to get the project in place. In many instances this resulted in hidden costs for the organisation which either had to re-advertise the job, redefine the whole-time equivalent dedicated to the project, or cover additional costs within their own budget. The salary scale on which the project facilitator was placed frequently did not reflect the level of responsibility they were given. Many project facilitators invested a great deal of personal time in getting the project completed.

Recommendation 12.4

The proposals need to be carefully scrutinised to ensure that the funding request for the project facilitator realistically reflects the demands of the post. In addition, it would be helpful for trusts to be alerted to some of the hidden costs they may encounter, e.g. practice nurse time; steering committee time; attendance at conferences; travelling expenses; making resources available to ensure the clinicians could work according to the guideline; and administrative support.

12.5 Impact on practitioners

Face-to-face contact with practitioners was the most important interaction in order to get people enthusiastic about the guideline and the ACE project. Both the literature and the findings from this study suggest that it is important for the project facilitators disciplinary background to match that of the target practitioners.

Recommendation 12.5

The project facilitator's disciplinary background should match the target practitioner's background. Where there is a multi-disciplinary project, the project facilitator should co-ordinate a multi-disciplinary team representing each target profession. The whole-time equivalent of the project facilitator should reflect sufficient time to ensure one-to-one interaction with practitioners.

12.6 Learning support

The varied academic and professional backgrounds of the project facilitators meant that finding the right theoretical level and creating an appropriate learning environment to support the participants was complex. However, the facility of telephone consultation with the HCEU was highly valued by the project facilitators.

Recommendation 12.6

It may be more helpful for project facilitators to identify the learning support and at what level they require that input, rather than putting on a standard programme. Although every attempt was made to make the learning support days as informal as possible, sometimes the ambience of the centre was found to be imposing and this inhibited discussion.

12.7 Guideline development

The way in which the guideline was developed and then implemented affected the number of practitioners who were actively involved in using it. The different approaches included:

1 National guideline – adapted into an implementation tool

2 National guideline – distributed unchanged – broad professional agreement

3 Guideline developed locally – local consensus

4 National guideline – adapted slightly to incorporate local patterns of referral

5 Guideline developed locally – local disagreement

6 National guideline unchanged – local disagreement

Recommendation 12.7

There needs to be clear direction from the funder of ACE projects as to what they want from the initiative; be it a developmental or consolidating exercise on guideline work. If they are hoping to encourage the use of guidelines in areas with no past experience, they may encourage organisations to use approaches 1–3. However, if they are hoping to extend the potential of organisations with a well-established guideline network, that organisation might be encouraged to apply more ambitious approaches/topics, indicated in 4–6.

12.8 Education strategy

A key to the high, medium or low effect of the project in reaching a number of practitioners and getting them to adopt the guideline seemed to be embedded in the education strategy or launch event. Launches by seminar or conference were successful in attracting a number of people, had the advantage of being less labour intensive (unless repeated on a number of occasions), but only successfully reached people who were interested enough to attend. Specific strategies to make sure that change occurred as a result of the learning that took place on the education day (e.g. action plans that were audited) helped to encourage change but were additionally labour intensive.

The hardest group to get *en masse* were GPs. However, access to GPs was achieved more successfully when using programmed educational events or through one-to-one interaction with GPs in their surgeries.

Nursing groups were more readily brought together when the event was held away from the practice setting and when they were given formal permission or encouragement to attend the event.

Recommendation 12.8

When trying to assemble a group of clinicians together to launch the guideline or undertake an educational session, the culture of that group should be taken account of so that the educational event is tailored to match their educational norm.

12.9 Changing practitioner behaviour

The most effective means of changing behaviour and sustaining practice according to the guideline was achieved: first, by continued interaction with the project facilitator throughout the project; and, second, by ensuring the guideline was implemented in the form of a tool that was used by the practitioners. The least effective strategy for dissemination was sending out national guidelines by post when there was no local agreement with the guidelines. Even when this was, followed up by one-to-one interaction with practitioners it did not bring about a significant change in clinician behaviour.

Recommendation 12.9

One-to-one interaction (between the project facilitator and the clinicians using the guideline), although labour intensive, should be encouraged. Postal distribution of the guidelines should only be considered in extreme circumstances and then with reservation, as short-term financial savings are outweighed by the low impact on changing clinician behaviour.

12.10 Patient/client involvement

Patients and clients were used in two key ways: as a member of the steering group and to evaluate the impact of the guideline on their care or knowledge about their illness or treatment. In a few instances they were involved in the decision-making process about treatment regimes. This was limited relative to the broad proposals suggested in the literature.

User representation is still in its infancy and in some cases the representative was there as a token rather than a real and valued contributor to the process. In some circumstances the teams felt the guidelines were too technical for the user to comment on and in others the users felt that the guidelines were the business of clinicians and they had little to contribute to the discussion. When the guidelines were written for patients or clients, then the user representative was more actively involved. Using a patient or client in treatment on the steering committee had the potential to alter the therapeutic relationship between themselves and the clinician fundamentally.

Recommendation 12.10

Patients and clients who represent users of the service may be more appropriately chosen from a group of past patients rather than people currently receiving treatment.

Project leaders need to contemplate how they can use patients and client representatives in more creative ways in the project. It is most effective to use the patient or client when a guideline is written for their use. It is perhaps an ideal to suggest that they can influence clinicians' guidelines unless they are extremely articulate and assertive. This would then raise an issue about representativeness of the patient/client group.

12.11 Barriers

Many of the barriers encountered when implementing the project were the reason why the project had been set up in the first place. Inconsistent practice, context-related difficulties, communicating within and across multi-disciplinary boundaries, and across different organisations, were the key challenges which had to be resolved. Gaining the participation of disparate groups of workers and trying to get them to work within a standard system generated resistance. In some cases this meant that project objectives had to be reformulated or alternative strategies adopted. Additional demands on fundholders' money to purchase equipment caused some friction when this resource was not covered by external funding.

Recommendation 12.11

(i) Knowledge of the organisation and knowing the people who work there helps project facilitators identify resisters and barriers. An opinion leader, with sufficient positional and legitimate authority needs to be a member of the project team to work with more complex aspects of change management.

(ii) Organisations working with guidelines for the first time might well do better to start this type of work on less controversial topics or with a homogeneous work force. Only those who are consolidating guideline work should be encouraged to approach more complex and controversial aspects.

(iii) A more flexible time-scale for projects should be encouraged; one year for certain projects is unrealistic.

(iv) When, or if, guidelines are introduced that require an additional financial outlay, there needs to be agreement as to how that expenditure will be met and by whom, before the guidelines are introduced.

12.12 Access to senior personnel

All the project facilitators had either direct or indirect access to the Executive Board or senior managers within an organisation. Only one site felt the lack of Trust support for their project.

Recommendation 12.12

All project facilitators should have access to senior personnel in the organisation, either directly or through line managers. Having an executive on the project team might cause suspicion among clinicians unless that person has clinical credibility.

12.13 Levers

Significant levers included tapping into pre-existing systems within an organisation and using those systems to implement the ACE project. The following circumstances influenced the amount of time it took to set up the project. As one descends through the list, the project facilitator had to invest more time in establishing the networks and systems to aid the guideline process.

1 A pre-existing guideline development, dissemination and implementation network with board support.

2 A clear R&D strategy; Audit Department and board level support brought together to aid the project.

3 A clear R&D Strategy & Internal Audit Department.

4 Access to external R&D and Audit Department personnel.

5 Project managed by project facilitator without support of R&D personnel or the Audit Department.

Recommendation 12.13

The time and money given to a project should be based on a careful analysis of the project site and granted relative to the banding and complexity of the proposed project.

12.14 Clinical credibility

The project facilitator's clinical credibility, or vicarious credibility by association with an opinion leader, was influential in encouraging recruitment to the project and the pooling or sharing of resources. The importance of professional relationships and knowing the organisation cannot be underestimated in its value to effect change and enable practitioners to respond positively to an ACE initiative.

Recommendation 12.14

The profile of the project team should reflect an appropriate mix of people with different skills. The membership of the team should include practitioners who are clinically credible to the target practitioners.

12.15 Applicability of the guideline

The quality and applicability of the guideline was a powerful lever. Having a robust guideline which could be seen to have direct benefit to the practitioner and their patient meant it was more likely to be adopted, especially if the guideline was being advocated by a practitioner who had clinical credibility.

Recommendation 12.15

The guideline should be implemented in the form of a user friendly tool that enables practice and reduces paperwork (e.g. as a management plan, an integrated care pathway or an assessment tool).

12.16 Sustainability

Some projects were set up in the hope that funds would be made available to them once the ACE money had finished. Others saw this as a one-year initiative. When the project was associated with a key facilitator whose role was discontinued after external funding the sustainability of the project was doubtful.

Recommendation 12.16

The project bid should include assurances by the trust that some provision will be made to sustain the project if its outcomes are positive.

12.17 Succession planning

The fact that the projects only lasted for one year meant that success planning became a low priority. It was difficult for the sites to seek internal funding to continue their work because the annual process for bidding for resources occurred at a time when the outcomes of the project were not available to substantiate that claim.

Recommendation 12.17

The project plan should include some indication as to how the team will ensure the project is sustained, either through an explicit succession plan or by identifying measures to ensure the maintenance and review of the guideline after external funding has discontinued.

12.18 Retaining expertise

When a project facilitator was lost to an organisation this not only had an adverse reaction on the sustainability of the project, but also meant that all the collateral learning accrued from running the project was lost to that organisation.

Recommendation 12.18

Using project facilitators in post or seconded to a project (rather than external appointees on short-term contracts) would be more likely to ensure retention of skills, sustainability of the original project and diversification.

12.19 The buddy

The buddy system for the majority was unsuccessful. There was a lack of clarity about the role. Most buddies needed more guidance to help them with the role of facilitating others.

Recommendation 12.19

More attention needs to be paid to the preparation of the buddies. Specific aspects included: active listening; giving and receiving constructive criticism; and clarification over role boundaries. The first meeting between the buddies and the buddied needed more time, to be made more informal and to encourage more discussion.

12.20 Facilitation by buddies

The clinical and academic background of the buddies differed greatly, as did their experience of project management and teaching. The idea that experience of running one ACE project was enough to facilitate someone else doing an ACE project was unrealistic. Project facilitators turned to trusted colleagues to guide them with their project. Insider knowledge of the organisation and the practitioners working there was considered more valuable than contact with someone who had ACE experience in another organisation. All the sites stated they needed more explicit clarification about: the format of the final report; written outcomes and standards against which the project would be judged by HCEU.

Recommendation 12.20

A buddy/mentor should be identified from within the site's own organisation. That person should have sufficient knowledge of: project planning; change management; and facilitation skills. If an external ACE buddy is used, he/she should be matched for professional and academic compatibility and, wherever possible, by similar topic. More formal written guidance from HCEU is required.

Acknowledgements

We are grateful to all those involved in the ACE projects who gave their time so generously to talk to us, and to members of the HCEU facilitating the ACE Programme.

The Steering Group: Sylvia Wyatt, Steve Dewar, Susan Holmes, Carmel Keller, Ann Mulhall.

Lynn Harris, Senior Project Officer at NHSE South Thames and Ron Stamp, Research and Development Manager, NHSE South Thames.

The evaluation team

Professor Carolyn Miller BA (Hons) D. Phil

Professor Miller is Head of the Centre for Nursing and Midwifery Research, University of Brighton. She has considerable experience in research in psychology at Cambridge University and in the development of evaluation methodology at the Universities of Edinburgh and Sussex. She is currently directing a national, three-year project, funded by the FNB to study how multi-professional clinical teams work in the current context of the NHS and how this knowledge can be integrated into innovative developments in shared learning in higher education. She is also co-directing an evaluation of the impact of the Primary Health Care Team Training Programme in South Thames.

Dr Julie Scholes RGN DipN DANS MSc D. Phil

Dr Scholes is Senior Lecturer in the Centre for Nursing and Midwifery Research, University of Brighton. She has undertaken a series of research and evaluation projects examining the impact of innovation on patients, practitioners and practice in a variety of clinical settings (including mental health; community and hospital settings in both nursing and midwifery). She has a particular interest in the impact of change upon institutions, units and individuals as a result of innovation and or educational experience.

Peggy Freeman RGN DipN MBA

Mrs Freeman is the Assistant Director of Nursing and Operational Services at Worthing and Southlands Hospital NHS Trust. As part of this role she is responsible for co-ordinating professional development of nurses within the Trust. She has been involved in ensuring clinical effectiveness in settings both in the US and UK and has considerable experience of designing, conducting and monitoring clinical audit.

References

American Psychiatric Association (1997) Practice guidelines for the treatment of patients with schizophrenia. *American Journal of Psychiatry*, **154**: April 1997 Supplement.

Anderson HR, Butland RK and Strachan DP (1994) Trends in prevalence and severity of childhood asthma. *BMJ*, **308**: 1600–4.

British Thoracic Society (1993) Guidelines on the management of asthma. *BMJ*, **306**: 776–82.

Clinical Standards Advisory Group (1995) *Report of a CSAG Committee on Schizophrenia*, Volume 1. HMSO, London.

Cluzeau F, Littlejohns P, Grimshaw J and Feder G (1997) National survey of UK guidelines for the management of coronary heart disease, lung and breast cancer, asthma and depression. *Journal of Clinical Effectiveness*, **2**(4): 120–3.

Conway M, Melzer D, Shepherd G *et al*. (1994) *A companion to purchasing adult mental health services*. Sainsbury Centre for Mental Health, London.

Duff L, Kitson A, Seers K *et al*. (1996) Clinical guidelines: an introduction to their development and implementation. *Journal of Advanced Nursing*, **23**: 887–95.

Effective Health Care Bulletin (1995) *The Management of Menorrhagia*, Vol 1, No. 9.

Effective Health Care Bulletin (1997) *Compression Therapy for Venous Leg Ulcers*, Vol 3, No. 4.

Farmer A (1993) Medical practice guidelines: lessons from the United States. *BMJ*, **307**: 313–17.

Field MJ and Lohr K (1992) *Guidelines for Clinical Practice: from development to use.* National Academy Press, Washington DC.

Grimshaw JM and Russell IT (1993) Effect of clinical guidelines on medical practice: a systematic review of rigorous evaluations. *Lancet*, **342**: 1317–22.

Grimshaw JM and Russell IT (1994) Health gains through clinical guidelines II: ensuring guidelines change medical practice. *Quality in Health Care*, **3**: 45–52.

Grol R (1997) Beliefs and evidence in changing clinical practice. *BMJ*, **315**: 418–21.

Hayes S (1997) *Clinical skills development: a study of the training needs of community mental health care professionals working with people with schizophrenia.* BSc Nursing Studies Dissertation. King's College, London. Unpublished.

Henning L (1997) *Physical health needs of patients suffering with schizophrenia.* BSc Nursing Studies Dissertation. King's College, London. Unpublished.

Kendrick T (1996) Cardiovascular and respiratory risk factors and symptoms among general practice patients with schizophrenia. *British Journal of Psychiatry*, **169**: 733–9.

Mari J and Streiner D (1996) The effects of family intervention those with schizophrenia. In: Adams C, Anderson J and De Jesu Mari (eds) *Schizophrenia Module. Cochrane Database of Systematic Reviews.* Cochrane Database, Oxford.

Morrell CJ, Walters SJ, Dixon S *et al.* (1998) Cost-effectiveness of community leg ulcer clinics, a randomised controlled trial. *BMJ*, **316**: 1487–91.

Plumb A and Jeffries S (1996) *Extent to which two community mental health teams offer a full range of evidence-based interventions to people with schizophrenia.* Clinical audit report. Pathfinder NHS Trust. Unpublished.

Ritchie J and Spencer L (1994) Qualitative data analysis for applied policy research. In: Bryman A and Burgess RG (eds) *Analysing Qualitative Data.* Routledge, London.

Royal College of General Practitioners (1995) *Report from General Practice 26: The Development and Implementation of Clinical Guidelines.* RCGP, London.

Sackett D, Richardson W, Rosenberg W and Haynes R (1997) *Evidence-based Medicine: how to practice and teach EBM.* Churchill Livingstone, Edinburgh.

Scally G and Donaldson LJ (1998) Clinical governance and the drive for quality improvement in the new NHS in England. *BMJ,* **317**: 61–9.

Further reading

All projects produced reports which are available from the chapter authors.

DoH (1998) *A First Class Service: quality in the new NHS*. Department of Health, London.

DoH (1996) *Clinical Guidelines: using clinical guidelines to improve patient care within the NHS*. Department of Health, London.

DoH (1997) *The New NHS: modern, dependable*. Department of Health, London.

Index